NUTRITION AND DIET RESEARCH PROGRESS

MALNUTRITION

RISK FACTORS, HEALTH EFFECTS AND PREVENTION

NUTRITION AND DIET RESEARCH PROGRESS

Additional books in this series can be found on Nova's website under the Series tab.

Additional E-books in this series can be found on Nova's website under the E-book tab.

NUTRITION AND DIET RESEARCH PROGRESS

MALNUTRITION

RISK FACTORS, HEALTH EFFECTS AND PREVENTION

JOHANNA B. KNUDSEN
EDITOR

Nova Science Publishers, Inc.
New York

For permission to use material from this book please contact us:
Telephone 631-231-7269; Fax 631-231-8175
Web Site: http://www.novapublishers.com

LIBRARY OF CONGRESS CATALOGING-IN-PUBLICATION DATA

Malnutrition : risk factors, health effects, and prevention / editor, Johanna B. Knudsen.
p. ; cm.
Includes bibliographical references and index.
ISBN 978-1-62100-351-9 (hardcover)
I. Knudsen, Johanna B.
[DNLM: 1. Malnutrition. 2. Age Factors. 3. Risk Factors. WD 100]
LC classification not assigned
362.196'39--dc23

2011033103

Published by Nova Science Publishers, Inc. † New York

Contents

PREFACE

Malnutrition is the condition that results from taking an unbalanced diet in which certain nutrients are lacking, in excess, or in the wrong proportions. A number of different nutritional disorders may arise, depending on which nutrients are under or overabundant in the diet. In this book, the authors examine topical research regarding the risk factors and health effects of malnutrition. Some of the topics discussed in the book include metabolic disorders due to nutritional changes during the prenatal stage; malnutrition in the elderly; malnutrition in inflammatory bowel diseases and genotoxic effects of malnutrition and infections in children.

Chapter 1 - The mechanism through which fetal antecedents contribute to disease development is not known but likely involves a complex interaction between environment and genetics. Nutrition plays a key role in the health of the individual; therefore, the prenatal period, immediate postnatal period, and the first months of life constitute a critical stage in the adequate development of an organism. Genetic and environmental factors in the prenatal stage are determinant in the association with diseases during adult life. Several studies in humans and experimental models demonstrated that an adverse intrauterine environment alters growth and may condition the susceptibility to experience future diseases. The present study explores some factors *in utero* that are related to "fetal programming" and their implications during fetal and neonatal life, analyzing maternal nutrition, intrauterine growth restriction and the epigenetic mechanisms that interact with gene expression during development, as well as some physiological processes that regulate the mechanisms involved in eating behavior from the prenatal stage until adulthood.

Chapter 2 - Malnutrition in the elderly is a serious and still often neglected topic. Nutrition disorders appear more often in the elderly than in the young people. Nearly all elderly people over 80 years of age suffer from a certain degree of malnutrition. This is a specific characteristic of the old age, when body compositional changes with a physiological decline in the muscle mass and a rise in the percentage of fat in the organism appear. This process in combination with pathological conditions typical of the old age as polymorbidity, polypragmasia, loss of dentition, bad psychological and socio-economic conditions results very rapidly in the development of malnutrition. The risk of malnutrition development in the elderly is increased by a number of chronic diseases. Conversely, already developed malnutrition aggravates the course and prognosis of most diseases. Malnutrition is a complex problem affecting several organ systems; therefore when evaluating the nutritional condition no specific marker can be utilised on its own to unambiguously prove malnutrition and it is necessary to use a combination of different methods. When diagnosing malnutrition in the elderly, it is necessary to consider the fact that a geriatric patient differs from a young adult and therefore the methods used could have a certain limitations that one should be aware of, i.e. other levels for pathological values etc. Timely diagnosis of malnutrition in the elderly can prevent patients from worsening self-sufficiency and quality of life, increasing the risk of institutionalisation, prolonging hospitalisations due to increased rates of complications and increasing the treatment costs and mortality of geriatric patients. Patients are mostly not sent to examine the risk of malnutrition, but rather for treatment of its complications. The only solution is timely recognition of malnutrition, and the initiation of nutritional support. The treatment of malnutrition in the elderly is based on an adjustment of dietary habits, dietary measures and sipping.

This paper aims to present a comprehensive survey of malnutrition in the elderly including risk factors, diagnostics, health effects, treatment, and prevention and to indicate specific differences as compared with a younger population.

Chapter 3 - Malnutrition is diagnosed in 80% of hospitalized Crohn's disease patients and in 20-40% of outpatients with Crohn's disease, whereas ulcerative colitis patients usually avoid the severe complication of malnutrition because in most of the cases the small intestine is spared. Nevertheless, malnutrition can become prevalent in periods of severe clinical relapse even in ulcerative colitis patients. Several factors contribute to the emergence of malnutrition in inflammatory bowel diseases, with the inflammatory activity, duration of the illness or flares of the disease, the extent of the inflamed intestine and the function of the intestinal epithelium being the most important.

Decreased food intake, macro- and micronutrient malabsorption and increased intestinal nutrient loss lead to a state of nutrient deficiency and body weight loss.

Oral or enteral nutrition is by far recommended in terms of improvement of bowel function and nutritional status. Parenteral nutrition is indicated only in cases of toxic megacolon, ileus or partial ileus, severe malabsorption syndrome, such as short bowel syndrome and growth retardation in children and adolescents for the acute phase when oral or enteral nutrition is not possible, since parenteral nutrition per se does not lead to sustained clinical remission, fistulae healing or avoidance of surgery.

Chapter 4 - Depressed inflammatory immune competence is characteristic of acute (i.e., wasting) protein and energy deficits in pre-pubescent humans and animals, and a substantial catalogue of clinical and experimental information has grown up around this classic observation. Unfortunately, however, the conceptual underpinning for the subject has not kept pace. Thus, the inflammatory decline associated with acute malnutrition continues to be seen in surprisingly simplistic terms as a component of a generalized and unregulated process of immunological disintegration pursuant to weight loss and limited substrate supply. This paradigm reflects a view of the malnutrition-associated immune system as an isolated silo without reference to other physiological systems or to the endocrine governance of metabolism. Although sufficient to launch the research front of nutritional immunology, such an unphysiological model cannot stimulate a scholarly development of the subject to productive maturity. Significantly, therefore, a new and more sophisticated concept has emerged, stemming from the point of view that any physiological change associated with acute malnutrition represents an attempt to adapt and, thus, is a regulated phenomenon conferring benefits in the face of a limited availability of energy and substrates.

Endocrinological and metabolic evidence is available of adaptive attempts extending even into the advanced stages of wasting disease in both clinical and experimental settings. In turn, this information base provides a framework within which to incorporate a body of immunological findings that defies the prevailing disintegrative paradigm but is easily accommodated by a newly-proposed adaptive, or regulative, model. The critical immunological evidence derives mainly from experimental animal studies of acute malnutrition in its more advanced stages and centers on studies of several cytokines that play key roles in defining the fundamental character of immune competence. As a consequence the proposition has emerged that acute pre-pubescent protein and energy deficit stimulates an immunological re-orientation emphasizing a non-inflammatory and tolerogenic form of immune competence. Such an adaptation may reduce the risk of autoimmune pathologies in response to a flood of catabolically-released self-antigens, but would do so at the expense of an increased susceptibility to opportunistic infection. This proposition, dubbed the Tolerance Model, provides a foundation both for renewed scholarly vigour in the study of malnutrition-associated immune competence and for optimism with respect to management prospects for the most debilitated clinical cases.

Chapter 5 - The purpose of this study was to evaluate the relationship between malnutrition, bacterial infections and citogenetic damage. In order to obtain the frequencies of structural chromosomal aberrations (SCAs) in peripheral blood lymphocytes, the authors sample malnourished and eutrophic children with and without bacterial infections. Fifty infants concurrent to the Hospital Interzonal de Agudos y Crónicos Dr. Alejandro Korn, La Plata, Argentina were included in this study; 14 malnourished and non-infected (MN), 11 malnourished and infected (MI), 18 eutrophic and non-infected (EN) and 7 eutrophic and infected (EI). Children aged 1-60 months. Anthropometric and clinic evaluation were performed to assess nutritional condition. Before blood collection, the authors interviewed each individual's parent to complete a semi structural survey specifying age, dietary habits, bacterial diseases; previous exposure to diagnostic x-rays; and use of therapeutic drugs. After 48 hours, 100 cultured lymphocytes were analyzed per individual. Statistical analysis was performed by the Epi Info 6.0, through the Pearson $\chi 2$ Test ($p<0.05$). No significant differences were found in total SCA frequency between MN and MI (14.2% vs. 15.1%). In MN children the total SCA frequency was four times higher than that of EI ones (14.2% vs. 3.33% $p<0.001$), and eight times higher than that of EN ones (14.2 vs. 1.8 <0.001). As well, in MI children the total SCA frequency was five times higher than that of EI ones (15.1% vs. 3.33% $p<0.001$) and eight times higher than that of EN ones (15.1 vs. 1.8 <0.001). Meanwhile the total SCA frequency was two times greater in EI than in EN children (3.33% vs. 1.88% $p<0.05$). Results presented here showed an increase frequency of SCA not only in relation with malnutrition but also with the presence of bacterial infections. However the effect of malnutrition was more important than the other. It is difficult to discern whether structural chromosome aberrations are due to malnutrition per se, bacterial or viral infections, or all of these factors acting on malnourished tissues. DNA damage could be attributed to several reasons: severe deficiency of essential nutrients (i.e. zinc, iron, and vitamin A) required in the synthesis of DNA maintenances factors; decline of repair mechanisms; and/or the absence of specific substances needed to protect the cell against oxidative

DNA damage. In conclusion, mutagenic agents cause chromosomal changes more easily in an altered environment.

Chapter 6 - Alzheimer's disease (AD) is a degenerative disease of the central nervous system and its progression is often connected with a development of severe malnutrition. However, sufficient data on nutritional state and intervention regarding the progression of AD have not yet been available. The aims of the authors' study were: a) to describe the relation between the state of mental function and nutritional status in patients with Alzheimer's disease and in those with dementia of vascular aetiology, b) to assess the relationship between nutritional support and the improvement, or the maintenance, of the patients' state of health. Methods: 165 patients from 7 institutions throughout the Czech Republic were included in a two-year-study. Voluntary food intake was measured during the first year following which the patients with Alzheimer's disease were randomised into two groups. The study group received 600 kcal supplements to their regular diet whereas the control group continued on standard diet. The nutritional parameters using the Mini Nutritional Assessment (MNA), body weight, triceps skin fold and mental state Mini Mental State Examination (MMSE) and Clock Drawing Test were monitored every second month of the study period.

Our findings: a) the nutritional status (MNA) was significantly worse in patients with Alzheimer's disease than in the patients with vascular dementia. The patients with Alzheimer's dementia who died had been suffering from severe malnutrition during the last three months of their lives. b) There was discovered a significant decline of the mental functions in Alzheimer's disease patients also suffered from malnutrition. Nutritional support significantly slowed down the deterioration of the mental functions of the AD patients. Interpretation: Their study showed that patients with AD are more undernourished than patients suffering from the vascular type of dementia, in spite of similar voluntary energy intake. Nutritional intervention significantly decreased the progression of the deterioration of the AD patients′ mental functions as well as other complications. It is concluded, that dietary counselling and nutritional support in patients with AD is clinically important and reduces the impairment of mental functions.

Chapter 7 - Anorexia nervosa and bulimia nervosa are primary psychiatric diseases, which can be characterized by food intake problems.

Recorded history of eating disorders extends into the distant past. Starvation, receiving a reduced amount of food or modified diet has been part of many religious ceremonies and rituals, acts of protest or response to poor living conditions. Already in the 2nd century, Galen described the first symptoms of anorexia nervosa. In 12th to 15th century women starved to silence their sinful body and claimed to be a saint.In the 16th century, however, these women were alleged to be possessed by the devil, and women were victimized by the church officials.

In: Malnutrition: Risk Factors …
Editor: J.B. Knudsen
ISBN: 978-1-62100-351-9

Chapter 1

METABOLIC DISORDERS: IS THERE A RELATION WITH NUTRITIONAL CHANGES DURING THE PRENATAL STAGE?

L. Manuel-Apolinar[1]*, A. Zarate[1] and E. Tesoro-Cruz[2]

[1]Endocrine Research Unit, Centro Medico Nacional, Instituto Mexicano del Seguro Social (IMSS), Mexico City, Mexico
[2]Research Department and Animal Facility, Instituto Nacional de Ciencias Medicas y Nutricion "Salvador Zubiran", Mexico City, Mexico, Immunology Research Unit, Centro Medico Nacional, Instituto Mexicano del Seguro Social (IMSS), Mexico City

ABSTRACT

The mechanism through which fetal antecedents contribute to disease development is not known but likely involves a complex interaction between environment and genetics. Nutrition plays a key role in the health of the individual; therefore, the prenatal period, immediate postnatal period, and the first months of life constitute a critical stage in the adequate development of an organism. Genetic and environmental factors in the prenatal stage are determinant in the association with

---

* Corresponding author: E-mail letymanu@yahoo.com.mx.

diseases during adult life. Several studies in humans and experimental models demonstrated that an adverse intrauterine environment alters growth and may condition the susceptibility to experience future diseases. The present study explores some factors *in utero* that are related to "fetal programming" and their implications during fetal and neonatal life, analyzing maternal nutrition, intrauterine growth restriction and the epigenetic mechanisms that interact with gene expression during development, as well as some physiological processes that regulate the mechanisms involved in eating behavior from the prenatal stage until adulthood.

Keywords: nutrition fetal, brain development, eating behavior, fetal programming, obesity

INTRODUCTION

Nutrition has crucial importance during the first stages of life because it influences an individual's growth and development, marking the predisposition to future diseases in adulthood. The term "programming" has been used to describe the process by which stimuli or nutritional manipulation exerted during critical or decisive stages of development that may cause short-, medium- or long-term changes either in the structure or function of the organism, with a possible compromise of health. Fetal programming was first studied in the 1970s and, during that time, the notion that not only genetics influenced the life and health of an individual was already taken into consideration [1, 2]. Nutritional alterations during pregnancy generate important changes in the organism of the future adult, affecting several metabolic, endocrinological, and neurological mechanisms. In fact, in a study reported by Barker *et al*, demonstrated a correlation between low birth weight (LBW) resulting from intrauterine growth retardation (IUGR) is one of the major causes of perinatal morbidity and increased risk of further adverse health outcome in adulthood such as obesity and chronic diseases [3]. On the other hand, the hypothesis that maternal anxiety or stress affects the neurodevelopment of the organism during pregnancy has long been considered, but it is only recently that detailed studies have been performed [4]. During the last 20 years, a series of studies allowed the understanding of the mechanisms by which such an effect is produced, and the findings have caused significant changes in perinatal psychiatry. For example, for decades the effects of postpartum depression in development of the newborn were not taken into consideration. It has now been observed that the effect of maternal anxiety during pregnancy is probably more serious and long lasting in the newborn than originally considered and that its neurodevelopment effects are more severe than those of postpartum depression. Several studies confirmed that maternal stress during fetal development may condition emotional and behavioral development, even up to adulthood. On the other hand, women of childbearing age should bear in mind the possible negative impact that psychosocial maternal distress may have on their lives and on the development of the fetus and newborn. They need to understand treatment options including social and psychological treatments, as well as possible medical treatments for these conditions [4].

This review identifies the effects of prenatal nutritional changes in relation to short- and long-term eating disorders (EDs) as well as to describe endocrinological and metabolic mechanisms. On the other hand, suggest some strategies that should be taken into consideration in the intrauterine life that may avoid ED's development.

Maternal Nutrition and Fetal Development

In previous times, maternal nutrition had considered that during the prenatal stage the fetus was exempt from damage due to external agents. It was supposed because the fetus was protected inside the maternal intrauterine environment. Optimal fetal growth depends on an efficient function of the placenta providing a suitable nutrition and gas exchange. This energy requirement is essential to stimulate growth and includes the active transportation of amino acids, protein synthesis, and steroid hormones. When placental insufficiency occurs together with maternal nutrition deficiency, it produces several effects on fetal growth. In addition, there is a decrease of substrates to the fetus, unleashing consequences that directly alter the metabolism of the placenta, diminishing its growth and affecting the transference of nutrients to the fetus. Thus, nutrition is essential during pregnancy and the neonatal period [5]. In current medical practice, nutritional care of sick neonates is considered a continuous challenge.

The fetus requires a series of metabolic substrates that can be grouped as follows: i) oxidative combustible for energy requirements that allow it to survive and ii) anabolic elements to achieve fetal growth. Prenatal malnutrition is an associated risk factor for metabolic diseases in adulthood. However, mechanisms of fetal malnutrition are currently unknown. This is an obstacle to understanding clinical problems in adulthood as a result of in IUGR, fetal macrosomy, and requirements of the premature infant [6].

Some studies determined that normal brain development depends on an adequate pregnancy and on the availability of oxygen, proteins, energy, and macro- and micronutrients as well as sensorial stimulation and social interaction after birth. Lack of some of the conditions previously mentioned or exposure to toxins (i.e., alcohol, tobacco, drugs, etc.) may cause disorders in normal development of the encephalon. The damage depends on the elapsed time from the onset of some of these factors in the nervous system to the time in which the process affects growth and development of the organism [7].

The encephalon grows at an extraordinary speed from conception until the third year of life, incomparable to any other developmental stage. Although growth and development sequences are guided by genetic information, the final result of brain development is determined by the interaction of this genetic information as well as along with environmental factors [8]. Maternal malnutrition during pregnancy causes LBW with a smaller cephalic circumference and brain weight compared with children born after a healthy term. These children usually have subsequent cognitive disabilities. After birth, breastfeeding plays a vital role in these children with prenatal malnutrition, benefitting babies and achieving, to a large extent, recovery in brain development and growth and its functions [9]. Some nutrients such as essential fatty acids (EFAs) are found only in breast milk and play a key role in the recuperation and development of a normal brain [10]. Research in premature babies has demonstrated that those babies who were exclusively breastfed presented an IQ 8 points higher than premature babies fed with formula [11]. However, prenatal protein malnutrition may result in a decrease in brain growth and in the production of neurotransmitters [12]. Even more so, it affects the myelinization process, which causes a decrease in nerve conduction velocity with neurons being the most affected cells along with the myelin-producing cells. In addition, axonal degeneration may occur [13].

In recent years we have learned that fatty acids are found among the most important molecules that determine the integrity of the brain and its capacity to perform its functions. EFAs are necessary to maintain an optima health status, but they cannot be synthesized by the organism and should be obtained from food. EFAs are extremely important for brain development, especially omega-3 fatty acids, both during the fetal stage and after birth [14].

In addition to their importance in constructing the brain structure, EFAs and their mRNAs are involved in the synthesis and functions of brain neurotransmitters and in immune system molecules. On the other hand, neuronal membranes contain phospholipids that are the reservoirs for the synthesis of mRNA lipids specific for neuronal stimulation or injury [14, 15]. These messengers, in turn, participate in the signaling cascade that may promote neuronal injury or neuroprotection. It is important to mention that the brain does not develop uniformly during the fetal stage and after birth. This growth has characteristic, well-defined stages, both from the anatomic and biochemical viewpoints. Neuro-genesis reaches its highest peak during the 14th week of gestation and is nearly complete during the 25th week, the time at which the total number of adult neurons is present [16].

Recent discoveries in mammals indicate that a limited period of vulnerability exists towards malnutrition. During that period, malnutrition induced brain damage and may have a limit effect in neurodevelopment potential [12]. Until recently, it was considered that alterations caused by malnutrition were irreversible, which has been refuted by recent studies demonstrating that the brain may possess an important recuperation process from the damages caused by early malnutrition. However, the remaining abnormalities include a reduced number of cortical dendritic cells in spinal synapses, reduction of brain myelin, and increase of mitochondria in cortical neurons [17].

O'Donnell and Grippo described that short apical dendrites, few spines, and anomalies in dendritic spines were found in infants with severe malnutrition and those alterations in the neurotransmitters seem to persist independently of nutritional recuperation. Among newborns with IUGR, only those with poor intrauterine cephalic growth presented neurodevelopment retardation after birth [18]. Also, exposure to nutritional deficiencies during the fetal stage has also been considered as a risk factor for the development of determined psychiatric disorders such as schizophrenia or bipolar disorder [19, 20]. One of the brain areas being specifically targeted in malnutrition studies is the cerebellum because its vulnerability to early malnutrition has been demonstrated. Some alterations of the cerebellum are irreversible, e.g., granular reduction [9]. Likewise, it has been determined that disorders developing in the central nervous system (CNS) during the first half of pregnancy affect cytogenesis and hystogenesis. The processes of growth and cell differentiation are affected during the second half of pregnancy and during the postnatal period. During the first 2 years of life, prenatal malnutrition may decrease brain growth. Another, important factor is constituted by the most important clinical sign of malnutrition, cephalic circumference [21]. However, the minimum amount of specific nutrients necessary for normal brain growth and prenatal development is unknown. On the other hand, it is also not known what degree of overall malnutrition is necessary to cause long-term alterations, cell irreversibility and neuronal connections. Children with chronic malnutrition more frequently present with anxiety disorders, attention deficit, cognitive deficits, posttraumatic stress, chronic fatigue syndrome and depression, among other psychopathological manifestations. These may be considered as a risk factor for EDs such as obesity, anorexia nervosa (AN), and bulimia nervosa (BN) [22]. Similarly, dietary restriction of essential amino acids may condition the correct balance in the production of neurotransmitters, affecting or modifying those systems [12]. For example, tryptophan and tyrosine are essential amino acids for serotonin, dopamine, noradrenalin, and adrenalin synthesis. Tryptophan is transported to the brain by a competitive brain system, which is shared with other neutral amino acids such as tyrosine, phenylalanine, leucine, isoleucine, and valine [23]. Psychosocial variations such as a change in tryptophan in the plasmatic concentration of one or more of its competitors directly modify tryptophan absorption in the brain. These variations in tryptophan levels influence the absorbance of brain tryptophan and, in consequence, synthesis of serotonin [23]. Serotonin plays an important role in brain development and is a modulator of cell proliferation within the neuroepithelium. It is also involved in different sensorial, motor, and memory functions in combination with cholinergic systems. A carbohydrate-rich diet increases tryptophan and carbohydrate levels in the brain and reduces tyrosine, making evident diet modulation in neurotransmitter levels, possibly explaining the behavioral changes observed in stressful situations in nutritionally deficient patients [24]. Other neurotransmitters contain amino acids as the basis of their synthesis, e.g., gamma-amino butyric acid (GABA), glutamate, and glycine, but their direct relation with nutrition is not specifically known. Some authors have described the importance of these acids in neuroprotection and in adequate brain organization [24, 25].

Fetal Programming, Metabolism and Feeding Disorders

The hypothesis about of adult diseases in relation with a fetal or early origin was proposed by Barker, he and his colleagues reported that environmental factors, mainly nutrition, acted in the early stages of life and programmed risks for the child to develop metabolic and heart diseases during adulthood [1]. During recent decades, several researchers suggested that the events implicated in normal fetal development have long-term effects and influence adult health. For instance, Fontana *et al* proposed that low birth weight infants were at increased risk for developing obesity, hypertension, and type 2 diabetes. Moreover, obesity is associated with impaired function of most organ systems, serious medical diseases, and premature mortality [25].

On the other hand, Hales *et al.* evaluated glucose tolerance in 64-year-old individuals and the results showed a strong association between LBW and metabolic diseases. Neonates with birth weight <2500 g had 7.5 times predisposition to develop diabetes or glucose intolerance compared with neonates who weighed >4000 g. So, that report was considered the origin of the "thrifty" genotype-phenotype saver theory [26]. Nowadays, prevalence of obesity has increased markedly over the last several decades around the world. But, there is a well recognized epidemic of adult obesity in United States, current data indicate that >20% of adults are clinically obese (body mass index ≥30 kg/m2), and an additional 30% are overweight (body mass index ≥25 kg/m2), and 15% of children and adolescents are obese [27].

The adverse health consequences associated with obesity include cardiovascular disease [28]; stroke; type 2 diabetes mellitus [29]; hypertension; dyslipidemia; cancers of the breast, endometrium, prostate, and colon; gallbladder disease; osteoarthritis, respiratory problems, including asthma [30] and sleep apnea; and perhaps depression [31-33]. So, there is evidence that early postnatal growth acceleration, which would normally be considered desirable, may exacerbate metabolic dysfunction in later life [34].

Excessive calorie intake and subsequent obesity increases the risk of developing chronic disease and decreases life expectancy. Likewise, if the degree of nutrient enhancement during the newborn period may modulate programming of appetite regulating hormones and neurotransmitters, body composition, and propensity to adult obesity in underdesnutrition newborns. In rodent models, calorie restriction with adequate nutrient intake decreases the risk of developing chronic disease and extends maximum life span [25].

Currently, new factors that interact with gene expression during intrauterine life are known and establish physiological and structural patterns with survival of the individual. Some of these not only influence the individual but also produce effects that alter the programming of future generations [1, 6]. The alteration in the availability of nutrients during pregnancy results in an adaptation during fetal development. This is achieved by metabolic, hormonal and neurological adjustments in the fetus with the intention of the newborn to be better prepared for an adverse environment (malnutrition). However, adequate nutritional intake after birth allows growth acceleration, possibly being the origin of metabolic alterations that may confer susceptibility of the individual to develop abnormal physiological functions and diseases in adulthood [35].

Thus, the environment encountered during fetal life and infancy appears to be strongly related to risk of non-communicable diseases in adult life. In order to explain these apparently causal relationships, there is an idea that propose that adaptations during critical phases of growth and development may ensure the maintenance of homeostasis, and hence survival, when the environment is compromised. A combination of genetic and both pre- and postnatal environmental causes is likely. In addition, adiposity is directly associated with offspring birth weight, with stronger associations for the mother and for the father, implicating prenatal environmental factors [36, 37, 38]. During the early months of life, when feeding patterns are strongly influenced by the infant and growth is regulated by nutrition, inherent patterns of increased or decreased appetite and satiety may return the infant towards its genetic growth trajectory. However, these patterns of early postnatal growth also appear to have more long lasting effects. In experimental studies exploring the "thrifty phenotype" hypothesis in animal models have indicated that long term obesity and disease risk markers can indeed be programmed by alterations in maternal nutrition such as protein restriction [39, 40], or by reduced nutritional supply to the fetus by uterine artery ligation in late pregnancy with □-cell secretory dysfunction [41-42].

Also, the energy homeostasis preservation requires intact serotonergic signals, some studies have determined that leptin increases the serotonin (5-hydroxytryptamine, 5-HT) turnover implying that at least part of the 5-HT effect on weight loss is mediated by 5-HT by increasing the serotonin signal just as this aminergic system seems to inhibit NPY system [43]. Some studies in mice demonstrated that alimentary modifications such as the administration of methyl donor compounds (betaine, B12, choline and folic acid) modified gene expression. Currently, a review of epigenetic markers in human nutrition is being investigated [35, 44]. Other studies determined that the development of the limbic system and the prefrontal cortex may also be affected by prenatal anxiety and stress. This appears to support the hypothesis of fetal programming, according to which some brain structures such as the hypothalamus would be programmed for adulthood during critical weeks of the third trimester of pregnancy. Similarly, maternal stress during those weeks may have permanent consequences, and the long-term magnitude of the effect could be significant [45].

In regard to the aforementioned, development of interventional programs targeted to prevent and decrease stress and anxiety in pregnant women is needed, along with prevention, detection and treatment of such situations [45]. The first studies on the effect of stress and anxiety during pregnancy were focused on observing the consequences of stress in obstetric results. It is known that women with stress conditions during the first trimester have a higher risk of miscarriage or their child may have congenital alterations due to a developmental alteration in the neural crest. An example might be cleft palate. The most well-known effects of maternal stress are premature birth and LBW [46, 47, 48]. Eating disorders such as BN and AN create the necessity for performing a neurological follow-up in a given population (bulimic or anorexic) to determine the vulnerability features of this group either by environmental or physical alterations. Recently, a relationship has been established between children with pre-, peri-, or postnatal history and risk of developing neurological problems [49]. Some studies performed in laboratory animals model demonstrated that the relationship between prenatal stress and behavioral adaptation alterations and emotional reactivity is strong and that such effects persist until adulthood. Alterations produced by prenatal stress in animals are diverse and not only related to behavioral and emotional disorders but also include cognitive, neurological and atypical sexual behavior [50].

Deminiere *et al.* observed in an experimental model that prenatal stress may alter physical and psychomotor development in animal offspring. It may also influence their exploratory behavior towards new situations during stress and, in general, in their social and sexual behaviors. Results of this study demonstrated that offspring from mothers stressed during pregnancy showed less interest in exploring a new situation [51]. Also, the relationship among the emotional status of the mother, fetal behavior, and variability of fetal cardiac frequency has been studied. Higher maternal stress results in less reactivity of fetal cardiac frequency, which may favor an inhibited behavior during childhood [51].

The main prospective studies regarding the effects of maternal anxiety on child behavior have been focused on a significant association between maternal anxiety during the third trimester and behavioral alterations and emotional problems during early infancy. Therefore, a direct relationship between the mother's emotional status and fetal behavior has been proven and observed in echograms during the 27th or 28th weeks of pregnancy. Several independent prospective studies found a relation between prenatal maternal anxiety and cognitive, behavioral, and emotional alterations in the offspring [52]. This relationship continues even after controlling the effect of postpartum depression and other variables in pregnancy and during the postpartum. A more recent study in newborns of mothers with anxiety showed that babies spent more time sleeping and less time being active and also had more mood swings [53].

Other studies performed at the Utrecht University (The Netherlands) in which 230 nulliparous pregnant women were evaluated from the 15th week of pregnancy until the first months of life of the newborn used several psychometric tests as well as maternal saliva swabs to study cortisol concentration. The results showed a significant correlation between fear of childbirth, fear of having a sick child, and stress with the decrease of the affective process of infants at 3 and 8 months of age. Likewise, maternal cortisol level at 24 weeks of pregnancy predicted alterations in the infants' adaptation processes at the same age. A strong fear of childbirth during the second half of the pregnancy was associated with a decrease of up to 8 points on the mental and motor development scale at 8 months of age. The negative effect of maternal stress during pregnancy was more visible at 8 months of age than at 3 months of age. It is during this age when babies begin to show interest in their surroundings [24].

Prenatal Nutrition and Their Relation with Feeding Behavior Disorders

The consequences of environmental changes (stress, nutrition) during the pre- and postnatal stage are determinant to learn if they are associated with EDs. It is known that EDs are chronic and progressive diseases, actually consist of a complex range of symptoms among which an alteration or distortion of body self-image prevails, along with a heightened fear of gaining weight. EDs are a mental health issue and are becoming more and more common among young women. If it is true that disorders defined by the Diagnostic and Statistical Manual of Mental Disorders (DSM-IV) such as AN, BN, and non-specified ED have a prevalence of merely 0.5 to 3%, then risky eating behaviors are much more frequent [54]. There is no unified concept regarding risky behaviors, but this term, as well as partial syndromes, abnormal eating behaviors, and subclinical disorders make reference to all those manifestations similar in context but less frequent and intense than EDs [4, 49].

Prevalence or incidence from EDs varies, depending on the size and age of each studied group, as well as the evaluation method [55, 56]. Studies in the U.S. and in Western Europe found an average prevalence rate of 0.3% for anorexia, 1% for bulimia in young women, and 0.1% for bulimia in young men [57]. EDs are presented with a M:F ratio of 1:6/1:19. Regarding the incidence of anorexia, the overall prevalence is at least 8/100,000 persons/year and for bulimia is 12/100,000 persons/year. For women 15 to 24 years of age, the incidence has increased since the last century [57-60].

Bulimia may present as a long-term condition fluctuating during several years or may be an episodic health problem, emerging as a consequence of life events or crisis of those who experience the disorder. In the short term, some reports suggest that there is a 50% improvement in behavior (binge and purge) in those patients who are able to commit to treatment. In this way, growth and development of an individual is a continuous phenomenon that begins with conception and culminates during the end of puberty, a period in which physical, psychosocial and reproductive maturity is reached. This transformation involves changes in size, spatial organization, and functional differentiation of tissues and organs. The relationship between nutrition and perinatal growth and the risk of experiencing certain types of degenerative diseases in adulthood is presently raising considerable interest [61]. Fetal programming may be shifted by the alteration of one or several relevant pathways during embryonic development or during the perinatal period due to nutrient restriction. Some of these alterations not only influence the subject but also produce effects that alter the programming of future generations. Other factors, such as drug addiction, alcoholism or ED (bulimia/anorexia) in the pregnant mother, cause fetal malnutrition [62, 63].

The term "anorexia" for some parents constitutes an alarm sign, probably due to its association with AN in teenagers, and the changing clinical data that may lead to other implications, both psychiatric and somatic. However, during childhood, loss of appetite may be due to organic diseases, either acute (e.g., cold) or chronic (e.g., digestive diseases). There may also be anorexia due to psychogenic causes, simple or transitory, as when the child stops breastfeeding, the birth of a new sibling, or alienation with the mother. There are some types of anorexia such as childhood anorexia that may affect one out of every three children <8 years of age. A child suffers from childhood anorexia when there is persistent difficulty to eat appropriately or not enough to achieve a correct increase of weight. The disorder persists when it is systematically present every day for at least 1 month without involving an organic disease or significant mental disorder. This problem usually starts prior to 6 years of age and may last for long periods of time. When analyzing the causes for not gaining weight are linked with the loss of weight, only 20 to 30% of children present a tangible, organic problem that will not allow them to gain weight and >50% present social, psychological or familial problems. Together with psychological conditions, some of which are jealousy of siblings, and organic diseases such as teething or gastric problems, other factors may strongly influence the eating behavior of children without appetite, as, for example, personality [45].

On the other hand, BN is a pathology of eating behavior and is characterized by secretly eating large amounts of food in a very short time at least twice a week for 3 months, followed by compensatory behaviors (self-induced vomiting, use of laxatives or diuretics) accompanied by a strong preoccupation for body weight and silhouette. In general, in brain circuits involved in the regulation of impulsive behaviors seem to be less active in women who suffer from BN. The frontostriatal regulator circuits involved in this study are mediated by dopamine and serotonin neurotransmitters. Nowadays, serotonin has been highly implicated in BN, which is frequently treated with antidepressants known as serotonin recapture selective inhibitors (SRSI). However, there are few studies regarding dopamine in relation to BN. BN mainly affects females and investigators are beginning to understand the neurochemistry of EDs [54, 64].

Magnetic resonance imaging (MRI) results of 20 females (mean age: 26 years) who suffered from BN were compared with 20 age-matched female controls. Healthy controls activated the area of the anterior cingulated cortex more when they gave correct answers and the striatum when they gave incorrect answers [54].

A. Causal Factors of EDs

Currently, consistent factors that would allow predicting treatment results have not been identified. However, severity of purging effects may be an important indication for prognosis: electrolyte imbalance, esophagitis, and hyperamylasemia reflect the fact of how severe the purges were and may generate an unfavorable prognosis. In severe cases, the patient may die as a consequence of binging or may even commit suicide. On many occasions, the patient presents symptoms such as anxiety and often takes anxiolytics to reverse the symptom. Thus, it is not possible to mention a solitary factor as cause of an ED because eating psychopathologies are multifactorial. There is a combination of individual, familial, and sociocultural causes that play an important role in the development and maintenance of any currently existing ED. Even so, the factors themselves should not be considered as definitive and with different causes but rather as an agent that may cause a person to become more vulnerable to developing an eating disorder [54, 65].

Malnutrition and the effects of hunger aggravate the underlying problems and become a chronic problem. In regard to obesity, three meta-analysis studies found that risk of obesity in school-age children is 15 to 25% lower in children who were exclusively breastfed in comparison with those who received formula [65-66]. The tendency to a lower incidence of obesity in a breastfed child may be observed prior to school age [67]. Multiple hypotheses have arisen to justify these differences that range from nutrient content and non-nutritive substances such as bioactive factors to the manner of feeding, sucking, or child-mother interaction. A rapid gain of weight in the first 6 months is correlated with body fat mass and waist circumference in adolescence. This correlation is not related to the relative weight gain after 7 months [68]. It is well known that the average weight gain in nursing babies who receive formula is higher than those babies who are breastfed, especially during two stages: i) the first 2 weeks of life and ii) from the third month of age on; therefore, it is difficult trying to correlate these two findings. As a result, it is suggested that an organism is susceptible to a predisposition or is vulnerable to develop an ED as a result of a combination of environmental, genetic, prenatal and neonatal factors [68]. Also, individual, familial, and sociocultural factors that predispose psychopathologies of intake of food are detailed.

B. Genetic Factors

Genetic studies suggest that the contribution of genes is ~50% in the development of an ED and that AN shares a high genetic risk along with clinical depression. This evidence suggests that genes influence eating regulation, personality, and emotions, being important factors in experimental studies with animals, giving especial emphasis in the animal conduct.

Different types of rodents have been used to study anorexia, exposing them to different stressful situations or annulling different genes. In a study reported by Lewis *et al* in which C57/BL6 mice were used, a common factor was found for all mice genetically modified ([69]. Chomtho S. *et al* studied the effect of the cannabinoid agonists (delta 9- tetrahydrocananoide) and the inhibitors of the recapturing endocanabinoides (OmDM-2) were studied [70]. In general, these types of studies suggest that the hypothalamic-pituitary-*adrenal* axis may be a related factor, although the results have been challenged because it is the investigator was who restricted the food and not the animal itself. Furthermore, it is not possible to consider cultural and social factors. However, cellular systems and mechanisms involved in eating behavior may be determined by this process [70].

Although hyperactivity may be considered as a strategy to lose weight, studies in animal models demonstrated that it may be explained using more complex mechanisms [69]. There is a strong correlation between serotonin and mood, sleeping, emesis, sexuality, and/or appetite (although it has not been scientifically proven). However, in a study performed in 2006, anorexia is related to a disturbance in serotonin, particularly those levels of the brain with the $5HT_{1A}$ receptor (related to anxiety, mood, and impulse control). Hypothetically, hunger is a response to such effects because it decreases tryptophan metabolism and steroid hormones, which may reduce serotonin levels and trigger anxiety. The complexity in these studies is that it is sometimes difficult to separate cause and effect because brain neurochemical imbalances may be the result either of hunger or of permanent features that may predispose a person to develop anorexia. There is no evidence, however, that some personality characteristics (e.g., anxiety and perfectionism) and serotonin imbalances remain after the patient has recovered from anorexia, suggesting that these unbalances are probably risk factors [71].

In recent years, anorexia has been associated with a series of metabolic molecules, playing an important role in the regulation of the immune response. In this context, leptin, a hormone derived from adipocytes, has demonstrated to regulate the immune response under normal conditions as well as under pathological conditions. More specifically, it has been demonstrated that conditions in which the production of leptin is reduced (i.e., genetic leptin deficiency, anorexia, malnutrition) are associated with a higher susceptibility to infections. On the contrary, autoimmune diseases are associated with an increase of leptin and the production of pro-inflammatory cytokines. Leptin may represent the "missing link" between the immune response and metabolic function, as well as nutritional status [72].

C. Social and Environmental Factors

Sociocultural studies have stressed the role of cultural factors with promoting "thinness" as the ideal feminine figure in industrialized western nations, especially through media. A recent epidemiological study comprising almost one million Swedish residents showed that gender, ethnicity, and socioeconomic status highly influence the possibility of developing anorexia. In this study, it was found that individuals with non-European relatives had less probability to become anorexic. Although AN is generally associated with western cultures, global media exposure has caused an increase in AN in non-western countries. However, it is important to point out that other cultures may not demonstrate the same phobia against overweight. However, another noteworthy feature among persons diagnosed with AN is an elevated rate of childhood sexual abuse (admitted by up to 50% of the patients, with a lower prevalence among persons treated in the community) [71, 72].

Neuroendocrinology and Food Intake

Thus, the degree of newborn nutrient enhancement and timing of catch up growth may modulate the programming of appetite regulating hormones, body composition, and neurotransmitters in CNS. However, in this period of growth may include aspects of enhanced orexigenic mechanisms (appetite), reduced anorexic mechanisms, highly efficient metabolism of substrates, and/or reduced energy expenditure. Experimental studies supports that hypothalamic control of appetite is likely set during the fetal or neonatal period, nutrient stress and perhaps nutrient enhancement during these periods may alter appetite set points. Prenatal stress (chronic variable stress) in mice experienced mid- to late gestation produced long-term effects on body weight in offspring from stress-sensitive dams, with male offspring being 15% heavier as adults at 6 months [73].

Bennis-Taleb *et al* have shown that exposure of the rat fetus to a low protein diet modifies vascularisation of the cerebral cortex [74]. Plageman *et al* extended this work and demonstrated that the early nutritional environment essentially hard-wires the brain to favour a state of hyperphagia. Besides, the common factor of a persistent of the hyper-phagia in animals exposed to fetal undernutrition or early postnatal overfeeding suggests that less than optimal nutrition at critical phases of development may promote adaptive responses that modify the areas or structures of key hypothalamic nuclei responsible for appetite control [75].

Therefore, the magnitude of the catch-up growth is conditioned by the interaction between genetic and environmental factors. In rodents, the impact of LBW due to early malnutrition results in catch-up growth inducing obesity. In study, we demonstrate that catch-up growth occurs in organisms following fetal malnutrition, but this weight gain induces obesity in adulthood. This process involves an increase in the leptin Ob-Rb expression in the hypothalamus. Thus, the results of the study further implicate the importance of leptin in the prenatal period and highlight that alterations in leptin Ob-Rb expression play a crucial role in determining long-term metabolic changes. Further elucidation of leptin receptor expression patterns during this window of plasticity will bring us closer to defining the precise role of leptin in developmental programming [76].

Vickers et al. indicated that severe fetal undernutrition-programmed hyperleptinemia leads to leptin resistance, hyperphagia, and obesity in adult life. Many of the effects of leptin on food intake and body fat storage have been attributed to its actions on hypothalamic neurons that coordinate behavioral and metabolic controls of energy balance [77]. All of these changes were amplified by postnatal hypercaloric nutrition. Also, several studies on rodents suggest that a defective programming of these hypothalamic circuits may begin *in utero* and continue in early postnatal life throughout the suckling period, leading to a disturbed organization and, consequently, long-lasting dysfunction in adulthood [78].

Likewise, dopamine receptors are associated with a variety of cellular functions in the mammalian central nervous system; dopaminergics receptor activation is critical for regulation of mood, motivation and motor function, including the feeding. Thus, dopamine receptors are coupled to G-proteins, typically, dopamine receptor activation leads to changes in intracellular cAMP levels. AMP-activated protein kinase (AMPK) is the downstream component of a protein kinase cascade that acts as an intracellular energy sensor maintaining the energy balance within the cell. The hypothalamus is a key regulator of food intake and energy balance, coordinating body adiposity and nutritional state in response to peripheral hormones, such as leptin, neuropeptide YY and ghrelin. Anderson *et al* studied leptin and they administrated it to rodents and founded that it lead a reduction in food intake, decreasing hypothalamic AMPK. These results suggest a relationship between dopaminergic receptor and peripheral homones, demonstrated that AMPK plays a role in the regulation of feeding and identify AMPK as a novel target for anti-obesity drugs [79].

Thus, dopamine regulates food intake by modulating food reward and motivation but its involvement in obesity and diabetes are much less understood. Recent evidence points to the involvement of leptin in the dopamine related modulation of food intake. Likewise, the importance of D2 receptor in normal body growth and growth hormone (GH) secretion in the neonatal period had been highlighted previous studies, and it alters the GH-releasing hormone–GH–insulin-like growth factor-I (IGF-I) axis [80]; an anatomical basis for an interaction of the dopaminergic and the GH system has been provided by colocalization studies, which indicate that a subset of GH neurons in the ventrolateral part of the ARC contains tyrosine hydroxylase, the key enzyme of catecholamine biosynthesis in rats [81].

Thus, if dopaminergics receptor expression in the hypothalamus is controlled by dopamine release, then by analogy to the basal ganglia, it is possible that an upregulation of D1 receptor mRNA in the VMH and a decrease in the LHA of obese rats could be due to a low or high local dopamine concentration, respectively. This hypothesis is supported in microdialysis studies, where were found differences in the baseline dopamine concentrations in the obese vs. lean Zucker rats [82, 83]. There are several possible explanations for the alterations, in other study D2 receptor levels compared between Zucker Obese (fa/fa) and Lean (Fa/Fa) rats at 1 and 4 months of age and in two different feeding conditions (restricted and unrestricted food access) using in vivo PET imaging and in vitro autoradiography, showed that D2 were higher at 1 month that at 4 of age and that food restricted animals had higher D2 than unrestricted animals. Thus autoradiography finding of an attenuation of the age-related loss of D2 binding corroborated previous studies of the salutary effects of food restriction in the aging process [84].

On the other hand, serotonin regulates different forms of synaptic plasticity both during development and in the adult brain. In particular, a major role for the serotonergic system is modulating learning and memory, mood and feeding has been suggested [85]. 8-OH-DPAT is a selective 5-HT_{1A} receptor agonist with a high affinity for 5-HT_{1A} receptors and 10- to 100-fold lower affinities for other serotonin receptors [86]. The affinity of 8-OH-DPAT for 5-HT_{1A} receptors is for p*Ki* =8.4 [87]. Centrally, serotonergic neurones in the raphe nucleus project to the hypothalamus and terminate around the NPY cell bodies in the ARC of the hypothalamus, and NPY-immunoreactive endings in the nucleus PVN [88]. Previous studies have suggested that some agents that mimic or enhance 5-HT action and which cause hypophagia and weight loss also inhibit NPY neuronal activity, although this is not the case for all such agents [88, 89]. Conversely, drugs that block 5-HT release or antagonize its action at 5-HT_{1A} and 5-HT_{1B} receptors stimulate feeding and NPY neuronal activity. This implies that serotonin may tonically inhibit the NPY neurones, and that the latter may mediate the effects of serotonin on energy homeostasis, this in the ARC; in this study suggest that is important to know relationship in the ARC between hormones and serotonin system in catch up growth, and impact in adult life.

Recent observations that people who develop coronary heart disease grow differently to other people during fetal life and childhood have, however, led to a new 'developmental' model for the disease. Low birth weight has been shown to be associated with increased rates of coronary heart disease, type 2 diabetes mellitus and altered glucose tolerance. These associations with low birth weight extend across the normal range of birth weight and reflect slow fetal growth rather than premature birth. The associations are thought to be consequences of developmental plasticity, the phenomenon by which one genotype can give rise to a range of different physiological or morphological states in response to different environmental conditions during development [90]. Central themes for prevention are the risk factors overweight, sedentary lifestyle, certain dietary components and perinatal factors. Overweight is the most critical risk factor, and should be targeted for prevention of type 2 diabetes, especially among children and youths. Ethnicity and perinatal factors are also worth considering. Today we know that prevention helps [91].

Thus, the phenomena of low birth weight as a result of nutritional perturbations *in utero* have been established in numerous studies [92], and its potential risk for adult diseases has been extensively demonstrated in humans and animal models [93]. But, in this study resulting phenotype has markedly different circuit neuronal suggested that announce in relationship with programming adult diseases.

CONCLUSION

In conclusion, maternal malnutrition has defined time windows with long term effects on weight gain and metabolism in the babies, besides, lactation is a critical period for the programming of adult life; suggest that in indeed, overfeeding immediately after fetal growth retardation induces a catch up growth.

In the present study it was our intention to review an issue not commonly addressed in neuropediatrics: the role of nutrition in the development of the nervous system. In the case of children with neurological or neuropsychiatric problems, it is imperative to perform an adequate nutritional evaluation to be able to detect possible cases, secondary to malnutrition or to a deficit of nutrients. Many cases may be reversible with appropriate and timely treatment because these patients are possibly susceptible for developing behavioral diseases that may have originated prenatally. Once the prenatal and neonatal factors related to EDs are known, we will be able to take preventive measures during penatal and early stages of life.

ACKNOWLEDGMENTS

We wish to acknowledge support of the Instituto Mexicano del Seguro Social and National Council for Technology and Research (FIS/IMSS).

REFERENCES

[1] Barker D. J. (1992). The fetal origins of diseases of old age. *Eur. J. Clin. Nutr.* 46, S3-S9.
[2] Lucas A. (1994). Role of nutritional programming in determining adult morbidity. *Arch. Dis. Child.* 71, 288-290.
[3] Barker D. J. (2004). The developmental origins of adult disease. *J. Am. Coll. Nutr.* 23, 588S-595S.
[4] Parcells D. A. (2010). Women's mental health *J. Psychiatr. Ment. Health Nurs.* 17, 813-820.
[5] Lucas A., Morley R., Isaacs E. (2001) Nutrition and Mental Development. *Nutrition Reviews* 59, S24-S33.
[6] Barker D., Hales C., Fall C., Osmond C., Phipps K., Clark P. (1993). Type 2 diabetes mellitus, hypertension and hyper-lipidemia (syndrome X): relation to reduced fetal growth. *Diabetologia* 36, 62- 67.
[7] Levitsky D. A., Strupp B. J. (1995). Malnutrition and the brain: changing concepts, changing concerns. *J. Nutr.* 125, 2212S-20S.
[8] Ropper A. H., Brown R. H. (2005). Normal development and deviations in development of the Nervous System. In: *Adams and Victor's*

"Principles of Neurology". Eighth Edition. Chapter 28. New York: McGraw-Hill Medical Publishing Division pp. 493-518.

[9] Bourre J. M. (2004). The role of nutritional factors on the structure and function of the brain: an update on dietary requirements. *Rev. Neurol.* 160, 767-792.

[10] Díaz-Arguelles., Ramírez-Corría V. (2001). Deficiencia de ácidos grasos esenciales en el feto y en el recién nacido pretérmino. *Rev. Cubana Pediatr.* 73, 43-50.

[11] Birch H. G., Pineiro C., Alcade E. (1971). Relation of kwashiorkor in early childhood and intelligence at school age. *Pediatr. Res.* 5, 579.

[12] Carney M. W. P. (1995). Neuropsychiatric disorders associated with nutritional deficiencies. *CNS Drugs* 3, 279.

[13] Mokler J. D., Torres O., Galler R. J., Morgane J. P. (2007). Stress-induced changes in extracellular dopamine and serotonin in the medial prefrontal cortex and dorsal hippocampus of prenatally malnourished rats. *Brain Res.* 1148, 226-233.

[14] Chang C. Y., Ke D. S., Chen J. Y. (2009). Essential fatty acids *Acta Neurol. Taiwan* 18, 231-241.

[15] Uauy R., Dangour A. (2006). Nutrition in brain development and aging: Role of essential fatty acids. *Nutrition Reviews* 64, S24-S33.

[16] Singh M. (2004). Role of micronutrients for physical growth and mental development. *Indian J. Pediatr.* 71, 59-62.

[17] Georgieff M. K. (2007). Nutrition and the developing brain: nutrient priorities and measurement. *Am. J. Clin. Nutr.* 85, 614S-620S.

[18] O'Donnell A. M., Grippo B. (2004). Malnutrition, environment and children's development. *Vertex* 15, 130-135.

[19] Pedrosa E., Locker J., Lachman H. M. (2009). Survey of schizophrenia and bipolar disorder candidate genes using chromatin immunoprecipitation and tiled microarrays (ChIP-chip). *J. Neurogenet.* 23, 341-52.

[20] Saugstad L. F. (2004). From superior adaptation and function to brain dysfunction: the neglect of epigenetic factors. *Nutr. Health* 18, 3-27.

[21] Ivanovic D. M., Leiva B. P., Pérez H. T., Olivares M. G., Díaz N. S., Urrutia M. S., et al. (2004). Head size and intelligence, learning, nutritional status and brain development. Head, IQ, learning, nutrition and brain. *Neuropsychol.* 42, 1118-31.

[22] Kajantie E. (2006). Fetal origins of stress-related adult disease. *Ann. N Y Acad. Sci.* 1083, 11-27.

[23] Fernstrom J. D. (1979). Diet-induced changes in plasma amino acid pattern: effects on the brain uptake of large neutral amino acids, and on brain serotonin synthesis. *J. Neural. Transm. Suppl.* 15, 55-67.

[24] Golubchik P., Lewis M., Maayan R., Sever J., Strous R., Weizman A. (2007). Neurosteroids in child and adolescent psychopathology. *Eur. Neuropsychopharmacol.* 17, 157-164.

[25] Fontana L, Klein S. (2007). Aging, Adiposity, and Calorie Restriction. *JAMA* 297, 986-994.

[26] Hales C. N. and Barker D. J. P. (2001). The thrifty phenotype hypothesis. *Br. Med. Bull.* 60, 5–20.

[27] Fontaine K. R., Redden D. T., Wang C., Westfall A. O., Allison D. B. (2003). Years of life lost due to obesity. *JAMA* 289, 187-193.

[28] Manson J. E., Colditz G. A., Stampfer M. J. (1990). A prospective study of obesity and risk for coronary heart disease in women. *N. Engl. J. Med.* 322, 882-918.

[29] Hu F. B., Manson J. E., Stampfer M. J., et al. (2001). Diet, lifestyle, and the risk of type 2 diabetes mellitus in women. *N. Engl. J. Med.* 345, 790–797.

[30] Chen Y, Dales R, Tang M, Krewski D. (2002). Obesity may increase the incidence of asthma in women but not in men: longitudinal observations from the Canadian National Population Health Surveys. *Am. J. Epidemiol.* 155, 191–197.

[31] Wolff G. L. (1987). Body weight and cancer. *Am. J. Clin. Nutr.* 45, 168–180

[32] Roberts RE, Kaplan GA, Shema SJ, Strawbridge WJ. (2000). Are the obese at greater risk for depression? *Am. J. Epidemiol.* 152, 163–170.

[33] Friedman KE, Reichmann SK, Costanzo PR, Musante GJ. (2002). Body image partially mediates the relationship between obesity and psychological distress. *Obes. Res.* 10, 33–41

[34] Eleftheriades M, Creatsas G, Nicolaides K. (2006). Fetal growth restriction and postnatal development. *Ann. N Y Acad. Sci.* 1092, 319-30.

[35] Lau C., Rogers J. M. (2004). Embryonic and fetal programming of physiological disorders in adulthood. *Birth Defects Res. C Embryo Today* 72, 300-312.

[36] Hernández-Valencia M, Zárate A. (2001). El peso fetal al nacimiento como factor de riesgo predisponerte para la diabetes tipo 2 en la vida adulta. *Ginec. Obst. Mex*. 69, 390-398.

[37] Hernández-Valencia M, Zárate A. (2003). El riesgo de diabetes gestacional se establece desde la vida fetal y posnatal. *Ginec. Obstet. Mex.* 71, 60-65.

[38] Bourre J. M. (2006). Effects of nutrients (in food) on the structure and function of the nervous system: update on dietary requirements for brain. Part 2: macronutrients. *J. Nutr. Health Aging* 10, 386-99.

[39] Petry C. J., Dorling M. W., Pawlak D. B., Ozanne S. E., Hales C. N. (2001). Diabetes in old male offspring of rat dams fed a reduced protein diet. Internation *J. Experim. Diabetes Res.* 2, 139–143.

[40] Ozanne S. E., Lewis R, Jennings B. J., Hales C. N. (2004) Early programming of weight gain in mice prevents the induction of obesity by a highly palatable diet. *Clinical Science* 106, 141–145.

[41] Jiménez-Chillaron C. J., Hernández-Valencia M., Reamer C. et al. (2005). □-Cell secretory dysfunction in the pathogenesis of low birth weight associated diabetes. *Diabetes* 54, 702-711.

[42] Hernández-Valencia M, Patti ME. (2006) Thin phenotype is protective for impaired glucose and related to low birth weight. *Arch. Med. Res.* 37, 813-817.

[43] Nonogaki K, Strack A, Dallman M, Tecott L. (1998) Leptin-independent hyperphagia and type 2 diabetes in mice with a mutated serotonin 5-HT2C receptor gene. *Nat. Med.* 4, 1152-56.

[44] Lee H. K., Park K. S., Deng J. H., Cho Y. M., et al. (2005) Mitochondria based model for fetal origin of adult diseases and insulin resistance. *Ann. NY Acad. Sci.* 1042, 1-18.

[45] O'Connor T., Heron J., Golding J., Glover V. (2003). Maternal antenatal anxiety and behavioural/emotional problems in children: a test of a programming hypothesis. *J. Child. Psychol. Psychiatry* 44, 1025-1036.

[46] Nepomnaschy P. A., McConnell D., Welch K., Strassmann B. I., Low B. S., England B. G. (2006). Cortisol levels and very early pregnancy loss in humans. *PNAS* 103, 3938-3942.

[47] Hansen D., Lou H. C., Olsen J. (2000). Serious life events and congenital malformations: a national study with complete follow-up. *Lancet* 356, 875-880.

[48] Hedegaard M., Henriksen T.B., Sabroe S., et al. (1993). Psychological distress in pregnancy and preterm delivery. *BMJ* 307, 235-239.

[49] Casasbuenas O.L. (2005) Seguimiento neurológico del recién nacido pretérmino. *Rev. Neurol.* 40, S65-S67
[50] Weinstock M. (2001). Alterations induced by gestational stress in brain morphology and behaviour of the offspring. *Progress in Neurobiology* 65, 427-451.
[51] Deminiere J. M., Piazza P. V., Guegan G., Abrous N., Maccari S., Le Moal M., Simon H. (1992). Increased locomotor response to novelty and propensity to intravenous amphetamine self-stimulation in adult offspring of stressed mothers. *Brain Res.* 586, 135-139.
[52] Di Pietro J.A., Hodgson D.M., Costigan K.A., Johnson T.R. (1996). Fetal antecedents of infant temperament. *Cgild. Development* 67, 2568-2583.
[53] Van den Bergh B., Mulder E., Mennes M., Glover V. (2005). Antenatal maternal anxiety and stress and the neurobehavioural development of the fetus and child: links and possible mechanisms. *Neurosci. Biobehav. Rev.* 29, 237-258.
[54] Field T., Diego M., Hernandez-Reif M., Schanberg S., Kuhn C., Yando R., Hoek H.W., van Hoeken D. (2003). Review of the prevalence and incidence of eating disorders. *Int. J. Eat. Disord.* 34, 383–396.
[55] Murphy R., Straebler S., Cooper Z., Fairburn C.G. (2010). Cognitive behavioral therapy for eating disorders. *Psychiatr. Clin. North Am.* 33, 611-627.
[56] Buitelaar J. K., Huizink A. C., Mulder E. J., Robles P. G., Visser G. H. A. (2003). Prenatal stress and cognitive development and temperament in infants. *Neurobiol. Aging*, S53-S60
[57] Rojo L., Livianos L., Conesa L., García A., Domínguez A., Rodrigo G et al. (2003). Epidemiology and risk factors of eating disorders: A two-stage epidemiologic study in a Spanish population aged 12-18 years. *Int. J. Eat. Disord.* 34, 281-291.
[58] Bulik C. M., Sullivan P. F., Fear J., Pickering A. (1997). Predictors of the development of bulimia nervosa in women with anorexia nervosa. *J. Nerv. Ment. Dis.* 185, 704-707.
[59] Lucas A. R., Crowson C. S., O'Fallon W. M., Melton L.J. (1999). The ups and downs of anorexia nervosa. *Int. J. Eat. Disord.* 26, 397-405.
[60] Yager J., Andersen A. E., Devlin M., Egger G., Herzog D., Mitchell J. III. Disease definition, epidemiology and natural history. Practice guidelines for the treatment of patients with eating disorders. http://www.psych.org/clin_res/quide.bk4cfm.

[61] Nielsen S. (2001). Epidemiology and mortality of eating disorders. *Psychiatr. Clin. North Am.* 24, 210-214.

[62] Favaro A, Caregaro L, Tenconi E, Bosello R, Santonastaso P. (2009). Time trends in age at onset of anorexia nervosa and bulimia nervosa. *J. Clin. Psychiatry* 70, (12):1715-21.

[63] Labayen I., Moreno L.A. (2006). Programación perinatal de la composición corporal. *Rev. Esp. Obes.* 4, 328-337.

[64] Berger M. A., Barros V. G., Sarchi M. I., Tarazi F. I., Antonelli M. C. (2002). Long-term effects of prenatal stress on dopamine and glutamate receptors in adult rat brain. *Neurochem. Res.* 11, 1525-33.

[65] Palmer R. (2004). "Bulimia nervosa: 25 years on". *J. Mental. Scien.* 185, 447–448.

[66] Harder T., Bergmann R., Kallischnigg G., Plagemann A. (2005). Duration of breastfeeding and risk of overweight: a meta-analysis. *Am. J. Epidemiol.* 162, 397-403.

[67] Owen C. G., Martin R. M., Whincup P. H., Smith G. D., Cook D. G. (2005). Effect of infant feeding on the risk of obesity across the life course: a quantitative review of published evidence. *Pediatrics* 115, 1367-1377.

[68] Armstrong J., Reilly J. J. (2002). Breastfeeding and lowering the risk of childhood obesity. *Lancet* 359, 2003-2004.

[69] Lewis D. Y., Brett R. R. (2010). Activity-based anorexia *Eur. Neuropsychopharmacol.* 20, 622-631.

[70] Chomtho S., Wells J. C. K., Williams J. E., Davies P. S. W., Lucas A., Fewtrell M.S. (2008). Infant growth and later body composition: evidence from the 4-component model. *Am. J. Clin. Nutr.* 87, 1776-1784.

[71] Meczekalski B., Podfigurna-Stopa A., Warenik-Szymankiewicz A. (2006). Anorexia nervosa--new view on neuroendocrine and genetic determinations. *Ginekol. Pol.* 77, 634-642.

[72] Matarese G., Procaccini C., De Rosa V. (2008). The intricate interface between immune and metabolic regulation: a role for leptin in the pathogenesis of multiple sclerosis. *J. Leukoc. Biol.* 84, 893-899.

[73] Mueller B. R. and Bale T. L. (2006) Impact of prenatal stress on long term body weight is dependent on timing and maternal sensitivity. *Physiol. Behav.* 88, 605–614.

[74] Bennis-Taleb N, Remacle C, Hoet JJ, Reusens B. (1999) A low-protein isocaloric diet during gestation affects brain development and alters

permanently cerebral cortex blood vessels in rat offspring. *J. Nutr. Aug.* 129, (8):1613-9.

[75] Plagemann A. (2006) Perinatal nutrition and hormone-dependent programming of food intake. *Horm. Res.* 65, (Suppl. 3):83–9.

[76] Manuel-Apolinar L., Zarate A., Rocha L., Hernández-Valencia M. (2010). Fetal malnutrition affects hypothalamic leptin receptor expression after birth in mice. *Arch. Med. Res.* 41, 240-245.

[77] Vickers M. H., Breier B. H., Cutfield W. S., Hofman P. L., Gluckman P. D. (2000). Fetal origin of hyperphagia, obesity, and hypertension and postnatal amplification by hpercaloric nutrition. *Am. J. Physiol. Endocrinol. Metab.* 279, E83–E87.

[78] Vickers M. H., Breier B. H., McCarthy D., Gluckman P. D. (2003). Sedentary behavior during postnatal life is determined by the prenatal environment and exacerbated by postnatal hypercaloric nutrition. *Am. J. Physiol. Regul. Integr. Comp. Physiol.* 285, R271-R273.

[79] Andersson U., Filipsson K., Abbott C., Woods A., Smith K., Bloom S., Carling D., Small C. (2004). AMP-activated Protein Kinase Plays a Role in the Control of Food Intake. *J. Biol. Chem.* 279, (13)12005–12008.

[80] Diaz-Torga G., Feierstein C., Libertun C., Gelman D., Kelly M.A., Low M.J., Rubinstein M., Becu-Villalobos D. (2002). Disruption of the D2 dopamine receptor alters GH and IGF-I secretion and causes dwarfism in male mice. *Endocrinology* 143, 1270–1279.

[81] García-Tornadu I., Rubinstein M., Gaylinn B., Hill D., Arany E., Low M., Díaz-Torga G., Becu-Villalobos D. (2006). GH in the dwarf dopaminergic D2 receptor knockout mouse: somatotrope population, GH release, and responsiveness to GH-releasing factors and somatostatin. *J Endocrinol.* 190, 611–619.

[82] Yang Z. J., Meguid M. M. (1995). LHA dopaminérgico activity in obese and lean Zucker rats. *Neuroreport.* 6, 1191-1194.

[83] Serguei O., Fetissov M., Meguid T., Li-Hua Z. (2002). Expression of dopaminergic receptor in the hypothalamus of lean and obese Zucker rats and food intake. *Am. J. Physiol. Regul. Integr. Comp. Physiol.* 283, R905-R910.

[84] Thanos P., Michaelides M., Piyis Y., Wang G., Volkow N. (2008). Food restriction increases dopamine D2 receptor (D2R) in a rat model of obesity as assessed with in vivo PET imaging [11C] raclopride and in vitro spiperone autoradiography. *Synapse* 62, 50-61.

[85] Buhot MC. (1997). Serotonin receptors in cognitive behaviors. *Curr. Opin. Neurobiol.* 7, 243–254.

[86] Hoyer D, Clarke DE, Fozard JR, Hartig PR, Martin GR, Mylecharane EJ, Saxena PR, and Humphrey PP (1994) VII International Union of Pharmacology classification of receptors for 5-hydroxytryptamine (serotonin). *Pharmacol. Rev*. 46, 157–204.

[87] Olivier B., Soudijn W., van Wijngaarden I. (1999) The 5-HT1A receptor and its ligands: structure and function. *Prog. Drug Res*. 52, 103–165.

[88] Dryden S, Wang Q, Frankish HM, Pickavance L, Williams G. (1995) The serotonin (5-HT) antagonist methysergide increases neuropeptide Y (NPY) synthesis and secretion in the hypothalamus of the rat. *Brain Res.* 13, 699:12-8.

[89] Boisvert JP, Boschuetz TJ, Resch JM, Mueller CR, Choi S. (2011). Serotonin mediated changes in corticotropin releasing factor mRNA expression and feeding behavior isolated to the hypothalamic paraventricular nuclei. *Neurosci. Lett.* (in press).

[90] Barker D. J. P. (2005). The developmental origins of insulin resistance. *Horm. Res.* 64, Suppl 3:2-7.

[91] Hussain A., Claussen B., Ramachandran A., Williams R. (2007). Prevention of type 2 diabetes: a review. *Diabetes Res. Clin. Pract.* 76, (3):317-26.

[92] Barker D. J. P. (1998). *Mothers, Babies and Health in Later Life.* Edinburgh, UK: Churchill Livingstone,.

[93] Gluckman P. D., Hanson M. A. (2004). The developmental origins of the metabolic syndrome. *Trends in Endocrinology and Metabolism* 15, 183–187.

This research was supported by FIS/IMSS
Disclosure Statement: The authors have nothing to declare.

In: Malnutrition: Risk Factors …
Editor: J.B. Knudsen

ISBN: 978-1-62100-351-9

Chapter 2

SPECIFICS OF MALNUTRITION IN THE ELDERLY

Dana Hrnciarikova[1], Bozena Juraskova[1], Miloslav Hronek[2], and Zdenek Zadak[3]

[1]Department of Gerontology and Metabolic Care, Faculty Hospital in Hradec Kralove, Czech Republic

[2]Faculty of Pharmacy, Charles University, Hradec Kralove, Czech Republic

[3]Center for Science and Research of the Faculty Hospital and Faculty of Medicine, Charles University, Hradec Kralove, Czech Republic

ABSTRACT

Malnutrition in the elderly is a serious and still often neglected topic. Nutrition disorders appear more often in the elderly than in the young people. Nearly all elderly people over 80 years of age suffer from a certain degree of malnutrition. This is a specific characteristic of the old age, when body compositional changes with a physiological decline in the muscle mass and a rise in the percentage of fat in the organism appear. This process in combination with pathological conditions typical of the old age as polymorbidity, polypragmasia, loss of dentition, bad psychological and socio-economic conditions results very rapidly in the development of malnutrition. The risk of malnutrition development in the elderly is increased by a number of chronic diseases. Conversely, already developed malnutrition aggravates the course and prognosis of most diseases. Malnutrition is a complex problem affecting several organ systems; therefore when evaluating the nutritional condition no specific marker can be utilised on its own to unambiguously prove malnutrition and it is necessary to use a combination of different methods. When diagnosing malnutrition in the elderly, it is necessary to consider the fact that a geriatric patient differs from a young adult and therefore the methods used could have a certain limitations that one should be aware of, i.e. other levels for pathological values etc. Timely diagnosis of malnutrition in the elderly can prevent patients from worsening self-sufficiency and quality of life, increasing the risk of institutionalisation, prolonging hospitalisations due to increased rates of complications and increasing the treatment costs and mortality of geriatric patients. Patients are mostly not sent to examine the risk of malnutrition, but rather for treatment of its complications. The only solution is timely recognition of malnutrition, and the initiation of nutritional support. The treatment of malnutrition in the elderly is based on an adjustment of dietary habits, dietary measures and sipping.

This paper aims to present a comprehensive survey of malnutrition in the elderly including risk factors, diagnostics, health effects, treatment, and prevention and to indicate specific differences as compared with a younger population.

INTRODUCTION

Malnutrition and deficiency states are found in the elderly very often independently of education, degree of information or economic situation of seniors [38]. In a higher age mainly the mixed, so-called protein-energetic malnutrition is observed [5, 40, 57]. There occurs mostly a combination of physiological changes in the regulation of energy input (a physiological decrease in energy consumption and total metabolic turnover, but with normal requirements for the consumption of proteins, vitamins and trace elements) with some pathological conditions and situations typical of the old age (polymorbidity, polypragmasia, loss of dentition, bad economic, social and psychic conditions etc.) [39, 40].

In a high percentage the senior suffers from malnutrition already before being admitted to hospital. During the hospitalization, nevertheless, there further intensification of the existing malnutrition often takes place and frequently malnutrition develops newly during the stay in hospital (the so-called iatrogenic malnutrition) in patients with the hitherto normal condition of nutrition [48, 87].

Good nutrition plays an important role in the care for the elderly, because it substantially influences the total condition of the organism–corporal as well as mental efficiency, resistance against infection, better stress management and more rapid healing of wounds. It also exerts a positive effect on the quality of life, decreases the necessity of hospitalization or institutionalization [80, 81]. In two thirds of seniors only an adjustment of dietary measures and dietary habits is sufficient to maintain a satisfactory nutritional state, only if this is not sufficient, some of the types of nutritional support is added [59].

It can be said that malnutrition and deficiency states are decisive for morbidity and mortality of the older population [9], because they represent a serious medical and economic problem and in a very substantial manner they change the therapeutic results even with the use of demanding and expensive therapeutic approaches [25, 58, 73]. Monitoring of the nutritional state and a rapid solution of malnutrition by introducing a good dietary regimen or nutritional support should be a standard component of both out-patient and in-patient geriatric care [4, 33].

Principal Characteristics of Malnutrition in the Elderly

Malnutrition and deficiency states occur very frequently in the elderly. This is a specific characteristic of the old age, when body compositional changes with a physiological decline in muscle mass and rise in the percentage of fat in the organism appears [22, 38, 50]. This process in combination with pathological conditions typical of the old age as polymorbidity, polypragmasia, loss of dentition, bad psychological and socio-economic conditions leads very rapidly to the development of malnutrition [39, 40]. Malnutrition worsens self-sufficiency of the seniors, increasing risk of institutionalization, prolonged hospitalization due to higher rate of complications, increases costs of treatment and also mortality of geriatric patients [6, 9, 37, 62]. In hospitalized geriatric patients with grave malnutrition, Duerksen et al. [15] demonstrated a statistically significantly higher morbidity versus the groups with mild malnutrition and with a satisfactory state of nutrition. Affection of the organism in malnutrition is complex and includes in a different degree all organ systems. The seriousness of their affection is due to the prevailing type of malnutrition [26, 38].

PREVALENCE OF MALNUTRITION IN THE ELDERLY

Disorders in nutrition take place in the elderly more frequently than in younger people; nearly every human being over 80 suffers from a certain degree of malnutrition. A more advanced form of malnutrition occurs in the elderly even in 50% [49, 86, 87]. This condition is usually independent of education, degree of information and economic situation of the individual [38]. Approximately 30% of older patients on admission to hospital suffer from malnutrition, which has been confirmed by the meta-analysis of Corish and Kennedy [10]. In 70% of patients admitted to hospital in various degrees of malnutrition, the degree of malnutrition deteriorates during the hospitalization [44], in 30% of patients with satisfactory states of nutrition malnutrition newly develops during the stay in hospital, i.e. the so-called iatrogenic malnutrition [48, 87].

PHYSIOLOGICAL CHANGES IN THE ELDERLY

In a higher age there occur some physiological changes in the regulation of energy input. Energy consumption and total metabolic turnover are decreased by about 10% [22, 41]. However, the consumption of proteins, vitamins and ions is not changed in the elderly. In spite of it, more frequently in the elderly patients we can find protein deficit, deficiency of vitamins and trace elements giving evidence of an insufficient supply of these substances in food in comparison with younger age categories [10]. This means that an old person mostly suffers from malnutrition already before hospitalization [40].

With increasing age there occurs a physiological loss of the volume of muscle mass by the so-called involution sarcopenia and replacement of muscle mass with fat tissue. Commencing with 40 years of age, 5% of muscle mass is lost in a decade and after 65 years of age the loss is even greater. Prevalence of sarcopenia at the ages above 80 years of age surpasses 60% [38, 87]. There occurs atrophy of the cardiac muscle, skeletal muscles (particularly the loss of the respiratory muscles is of special importance), as well as the visceral muscles [8, 13, 56, 64].

In the elderly there are also physiological changes in the gastrointestinal tract –loss of dentition, disorder is the motility of the gastrointestinal tract, deterioration of secretion of digestive juices, changes in the intestinal villi, atrophy of the intestinal wall causing deterioration of absorption of nutritional substrates with the development of hunger diarrhoeas and deteriorated capability of realimentation, increased risk of penetration of bacteria through the intestinal wall, decreased function of the pancreas, decelerated motility of the biliary tract, and a decreased activity of the liver [26, 39].

RISK FACTORS OF MALNUTRITION IN THE ELDERLY

A risk of the development of malnutrition in seniors is most frequently a decrease in the energy input or omission of some component of food (e.g. proteins). A problem can also be the diseases in which the patient loses appetite as the result of the health condition, or as the result of the administration of some medicaments. From this aspect, in seniors the most risky ones are chronic non-oncological diseases, in particular the diseases of the cardiovascular and pulmonary systems and the gastrointestinal tract. Also oncological diseases and their treatment significantly contribute to an increased risk of the development of malnutrition. In geriatric patients also long-term hospitalization can exert very negative effects. The problem is that in seniors very often the monitoring of the risk of malnutrition is not in the focus of attention of the health personnel [34]. The most frequent risk factors of the development of malnutrition in the elderly are listed below in Table 1.

Table 1. The most frequent risk factors of malnutrition in the elderly

Risk factors of malnutrition in the elderly
polymorbidity
polypragmasia
hospitalization
loss or defect of dentition, affection of salivary glands
diseases of the oral cavity, esophagus, gastrointestinal tract and liver
decreased appetite, bad dietary habits
involution sarcopenia, limited mobility
psychic disorders (depression, demention)
social isolation
insufficient stimulation and help of the surroundings
economic difficulties

Types of Malnutrition

Malnutrition can be generally divided into two types. The marantic type (the so-called mixed protein-energetic malnutrition) is connected with simple fasting. Kwashiorkor is malnutrition caused by a long-term deficit of proteins with a sufficient supply of energy, which is mainly the case of developing countries. Kwashiorkor-like malnutrition is due to insufficient adaptation of the starving organism to a disease and it develops if in a patient already suffering from malnutrition (simple fasting) a catabolizing disease (stress fasting) is manifested as a transition of the marantic type to the kwashiorkor type of malnutrition [38, 68]. This type of malnutrition is frequent in hospitals in patients in grave life-threatening conditions with insufficient nutritional support [10, 87].

In simple fasting in the early stage there occur activation of glycogenolysis in the liver, an increase in lipolysis in the fat tissue, and a decrease in proteosynthesis in the muscle tissue. In longer fasting after exhausting the glycogen supplies, fat becomes the principal energy source for the organism. The activity of tissue lipase and the wash-up of fatty acids into the blood circulation are increased. Fatty acids are employed as the source of energy in the tissues. In a smaller extent amino acids from the muscle tissue are then utilized. In simple fasting, an average decrease of 160-200g of fat (200-250g of fat tissue) and 20-30g of proteins (100-120g of the muscle tissue) takes place in a day.

In stress fasting, malnutrition and disease (the catabolic condition–mainly septic conditions, traumata, burns, extensive surgery, etc.) act simultaneously. There is marked stimulation of gluconeogenesis, in particular by converting amino acids from the muscle tissue. Amino acids are the principal energy metabolite in stress fasting. Up to 250g of proteins (1kg of the muscle tissue) are degraded daily [38, 73, 87].

Clinical Picture of Malnutrition in the Elderly

In the elderly there occurs very often mixed, the so-called protein-energetic malnutrition [5, 57]. Insufficient protein-energetic intake first results in a decrease in body weight. Energy is obtained from the fat tissue, later also from the muscle tissue [14, 19, 20]. After exhaustion of tissue reserves there occurs also a decrease in plasma proteins, which results in a disorder in the distribution of fluids in the interstitium and intravasal space with the development of swellings [37]. Furthermore, due to a decrease in the concentration of immunoglobulins immunological resistance of the organism is decreased with an increased risk of the development of infectious complications or even septic conditions, healing processes are decelerated with disintegration of wounds after surgeries with decreased proteosynthesis and prolongation of the convalescence period. The study of Brazilian authors [32] demonstrated a relationship between lower levels of prealbumin and transferin and a higher occurrence of infectious complications after elective surgeries, and they simultaneously found also a relationship between low prealbumin and the absolute number of lymphocytes and higher post-surgery mortality for infectious diseases. With a decrease in the muscles there is a higher tendency for falls [60], which with simultaneous acceleration of osteoporosis increase the risk of fractures and subsequent immobilization [68]. Weakening of the respiratory muscles results in hypoventilation and increased risk of respiratory failure [1]. There also occurs a decrease in the levels of cholesterol, vitamins (in particular A, C, E), minerals and trace elements (e.g. copper, iron) [21, 33, 74]. With a decrease in plasma proteins (in particular albumin, but also prealbumin and transferin) the transfer of the substances bound to them – hormones (e.g. cortisol), fatty acids, trace elements or pharmaceuticals (e.g. antibiotics) is also deteriorated [11, 29]. For instance, the efficiency of some antibiotics is also based on the balance between the ratio of the free and bound drug. With a decrease in albumin, there is also a decrease in its capability of binding the antibiotic, which in the free form is quickly eliminated and cannot thus reach the effective concentration [38, 46].

DIAGNOSIS OF MALNUTRITION IN THE ELDERLY

Malnutrition is a complex problem afflicting several organ systems therefore when evaluating the nutritional condition no specific marker can be utilised on its own to unambiguously prove malnutrition and it is necessary to use a combination of different methods (nutrition anamnesis, anthropometrical, laboratory and functional examination) with different predictive values [3, 17, 28, 43, 61]. The necessity of combining individual methods in malnutrition diagnosis in hospitalized patients is indicated by the meta-analysis of Corish and Kennedy [10], who also report the limitations of routinely used nutritional examinations. When diagnosing malnutrition in the old age, it is necessary to consider the fact that a geriatric patient differs from a young adult and therefore the methods used could have a certain limitations that one should be aware of, i.e. other levels for pathological values etc. [36, 42].

1. Nutrition History

Gathering a nutrition anamnesis should be an inseparable part of nutritional screening. We especially look for changes in body weight (see below). It is also important to identify dietary habits, dietary restrictions and diseases of the gastrointestinal tract. It is also pertinent to inquire about the use of vitamin preparations. Dental condition should not be overlooked in geriatric patients along with the influence of other concurrent diseases, cognitive functions, mobility disorders and last but not least even social factors as loneliness or lack of financial means [38, 42, 82].

Mini Nutritional Assessment (MNA)

MNA is a widely used international questionnaire to evaluate the nutritional state of seniors. This aid can select, with high sensitivity (98.9%), specificity (94.3%) and diagnosis accuracy (97.2%), the patients with a risk of malnutrition. It closely correlates with biochemical (albumin, prealbumin, transferin levels, and lymphocyte numbers) and anthropometrical markers (measuring of subcuticular fat, arms circumference) as it has been shown in the paper by Vellas et al. [84]. Performing the MNA is not time demanding, the complete form does not exceed 15 minutes and a shortened version can be filled in 3 minutes [83]. Performing a complex MNA is suitable especially in risk groups of institutionalised or hospitalized seniors. MNA itself consists of 4 groups of questions and measurements: basic anthropometrical measurement (BMI, arm, hip circumference, loss of body mass), total condition evaluation (mobility, self-sufficiency, chronic defects, presence of acute disease, psychological condition and polypragmasia), dietary habits (questions aimed at food and liquid consumption and the ability to eat) and judging the condition of nutrition and health. A certain number of points are allocated to each question; the maximum reached is 29 points, the minimum 0 point. Normal MNA and a good condition of nutrition is considered above 24 points, endangering risk of malnutrition appears in the range of 17 – 23.5 points and a score under 17 verifies malnutrition [23, 37, 79].

According to the Spanish authors Ruiz-López et al. [69], only 30.3% of older women from two houses for the elderly had normal values of MNA. The individual questions of the MNA questionnaire are listed in Table 2.

2. Anthropometrical Examinations

Anthropometrical indicators are simple, non-invasive and cheap methods of monitoring the state of nutrition and are especially suitable for out-patient monitoring. These measurements can help to reveal the extent of affliction in a given individual [38, 87]. The anthropometrical minimum for the purposes of nutritional evaluation is the measurement of arm circumference and the triceps skin fold [30, 33]. The study of Lasheras et al. [51] found a statistically significant difference in the values of the skin fold above the triceps muscle and the arm circumference in a group of institutionalized seniors versus those who lived at home.

Body Mass

Isolated measurement of body mass could be misleading, it is important to follow the values in time. Unwanted loss of body mass of more than 5% in one month or more than 10% from the baseline body mass after 6 months could reflect malnutrition [10]. A decrease of more than 10% in one month or more than 20% in two months testifies to a serious degree of malnutrition with an increased risk of infectious and postoperative complications, higher postoperative morbidity and mortality [4, 33]. In seniors weighing could be impossible due to inability to stand. In lying patients body mass and height could be estimated by special anthropometrical techniques. Unwanted decrease of body mass in the elderly, apart from malnutrition, could also be caused even by other diseases (tumours, serious cardiac and respiratory failures, dementia or depression) or social risk conditions (poverty and solitude) [38].

Body-Mass Index (BMI)

BMI is a basic guide to evaluate the nutritional state and the most commonly used mass-height indicators. Normal values of BMI are found in the range 20 – 25 kg/m^2. BMI under 18.5 kg/m^2 specifies cachexia, under 16 kg/m^2 grave cachexia, but in the seniors the risk is already under 20 kg/m^2 especially due to an increase of postoperative complications [3, 73, 87].

Table 2. Mini Nutritional Assessment (taken from: Vellas B, Guigoz Y, Garry PJ et al. The Mini Nutritional Assessment: MNA. Nutrition in the Elderly. Facts and Research in Gerontology)

I. ATHROPOMETRIC ASSESSMENT 1. Body Mass Index (BMI) (weight in kg) / (height in m)² a. BMI < 19 = 0 points b. BMI 19 to < 21 = 1 point c. BMI 21 to < 23 = 2 points d. BMI ≥ 23 = 3 points 2. Mid-arm circumference (MAC) in cm a. MAC < 21 = 0.0 points b. MAC 21 ≤ 22 = 0.5 points c. MAC > 22 = 1.0 points 3. Calf circumference (CC) in cm a. CC<31 = 0 points b. CC≥31 = 1 point 4. Weight loss during last 3 months a. weight loss greater than 3kg = 0 points b. does not know = 1 point c. weight loss between 1 and 3 kg=2 points d. no weight loss =3 points II. GENERAL ASSESSMENT 5. Lives independently (not in nursing home or hospital) a. no = 0 points b. yes = 1 point 6. Takes more than 3 prescription drugs per day a. yes = 0 points b. no = 1 point 7. Has suffred psychological stress or acute disease in the past 3 months a. yes = 0 points b. no = 2 points 8. Mobility a. bed or chair bound = 0 points b. able to get out of bed/chair but does not go out = 1 point c. goes out = 2 points 9. Neuropsychological problems a. severe dementia or depression = 0 points b. mild dementia = 1 point c. no psychological problems = 2 points 10. Pressure sores or skin ulcers a. yes = 0 points b. no = 1 point III. DIETARY ASSESSMENT 11. How many full meals does the patient eat daily? a. 1 meal = 0 points b. 2 meals = 1 point c. 3 meals = 2 points	12. Selected consumption markers for protein intake * at least 1 serving of dairy products per day? yes/no * 2 or more servings of legumes or eggs per week? yes/no * meat, fish or poultry every day? yes/no a. if 0 or 1 yes = 0.0 points b. if 2 yes = 0.5 points c. if 3 yes = 1.0 points 13. Consumes two or more servings of fruits or vegetables per day? a. no = 0 points b. yes = 1 point 14. Has food intake declined over the past three months due to loss of appetite, digestive problems, chewing or swallowing difficulties? a. severe loss of appetite = 0 points b. moderate loss of appetite = 1 point c. no loss of appetite = 2 points 15. How much fluid is consumed per day? a. less than 3 cups = 0.0 points b. 3 to 5 cups = 0.5 points c. more than 5 cups = 1.0 points 16. Mode of feeding a.unable to eat without assistance=0points b. self-fed with some difficulty =1point c. self-fed without any problem =2points IV. SELF ASSESSMENT 17. Do they view themselves as having nutritional problems? a. major malnutrition = 0 points b. does not know or moderate malnutrition = 1 point c. no nutritional problem = 2 points 18. In comparison with other people of the same age, how do they consider their health status? a. not as good = 0.0 points b. does not know = 0.5 points c. as good = 1.0 points d. better = 2.0 points

	ASSESSMENT TOTAL (max. 30 points) MALNUTRITION INDICATOR SCORE ≥ 24 points well-nourished 17 to 23.5 points at risk of malnutrition < 17 points malnourished

Mid-Arm Circumference

Measurement of the arm circumference is a simple method for the determination of the body mass quantity. It is measured on the non-dominant extremity at a site half way between the acromion and olecranon. Normal values are 29.3 cm in men and 28.5 cm in women, for a severe malnutrition with a loss of body mass testifies circumference smaller than 19.5 cm in men and 15.5 in women. It is suitable to combine the measurement of the mid-arm circumference and the triceps skin fold [87].

Triceps Skin Fold

Determination of the skin fold above the triceps indicates the quantity of subcutaneous fat. The measurement is carried out on the non-dominant extremity by a special apparatus called calliper. The normal value is 12.5 mm in men and 16.5 mm in women, the values smaller than 8 mm in men and 10 mm in women indicate significant malnutrition. In seniors this measurement may not be precise due to the loss of skin elasticity [87].

Determination of the Circumference of the Musculature of the Arm

It quantifies the loss of musculature by calculating the means of measurements of the arm circumference which is deducted from the layer of the subcutaneous tissue measured with a calliper upon the triceps. The normal values are 25.3 cm in men and 23.2 cm in women, the values of 15.2 cm in men and 13.9 cm in women testify for severe malnutrition [87].

3. Laboratory Examinations

Amongst laboratory findings, the current practise most often includes biochemical examination, where specifically a decrease in serum proteins identifies malnutrition [54, 63, 75].

Biochemical Examinations

Biochemical markers belong among the basic examination in the diagnosis of malnutrition. Formation of serum proteins in the liver is connected with the nutritional state of the organism, in malnutrition the proteosynthetic liver function is usually decreased. According to half-life of individual plasma proteins the duration of malnutrition can be determined [18, 42].

Levels of serum proteins decrease also during an inflammatory reaction (negative proteins of the acute phase) by a transfer of plasma proteins into reactants of the acute phase C-reactive protein (CRP), therefore it is suitable to determine simultaneously even CRP, whose value increases during inflammation (positive protein of the acute phase) and to mutually compare the measured values [10, 53, 71]. Low values of serum proteins in the elderly can be simulated by dehydration, after re-hydration a decrease in the markers occurs due to hemodilution [38].

Beside the values of plasma proteins even a low value of total cholesterol (less than 2.0 mmol/l) could testify for malnutrition and at present a possibility is discussed of employing serum lipids as biomarkers of malnutrition and possibly also of inflammation. Also a decrease of thyroid gland hormones can be a marker of malnutrition, a lower value of creatinine can demonstrate a low capacity of the musculature mass. These indicators must be evaluated with respect to intercurrently on-going diseases [54, 75]. Vitamin deficiencies in the elderly are usually very frequent; a knowledge of their levels is advisable in the adjustment of dietary habits and recommendation of possible vitamin preparations [85].

According to Sullivan et al. [78], in geriatric patients with more than a 50% decrease in food intake during hospitalization there was a marked decrease in total cholesterol, albumin and prealbumin versus the patients with the normal state of nutrition.

Total Protein (TP)

At present, total protein is practically not used as a marker of malnutrition. Its disadvantage is its long biological half-life, and therefore it is rather a late marker of protein malnutrition and provides only an orientational idea. Low levels of total protein may give evidence of a long-term protein deficit, but they do not demonstrate acute changes in the nutritional state. The physiological values of total protein are 65-80g/l, a decrease below 55g/l is considered serious. The value of total protein is usually significantly influenced particularly by hepatic or renal disorders, degree of dehydration, and a concurrent inflammatory process [27, 54]. According to Mühlberg et al. [60], a decreased TP value in seniors is a risk factor for possible injury.

Albumin

Determination of the level of serum albumin was formerly considered to be the gold standard in the evaluation of the nutritional state. At present, however, its role as a nutritional marker is doubted. Nevertheless, it is still a suitable marker for screening and long-term monitoring of malnutrition (if inflammation can be excluded); due to its longer half-life it is not suitable for monitoring acute changes in nutritional state. Its informative value is increased in combination with prealbumin, transferin or cholinesterase. A decrease in serum albumin level correlates with the total prognosis of patients, and it is an independent indicator of seriousness of a clinical state [27, 57, 87]. Kagansky et al. [37] demonstrate decreased albumin as a risk factor of malnutrition and in hospitalized geriatric patients confirm a higher mortality in malnutrition patients. The values of plasma albumin are also part of the majority of nutritional indices.

Albumin possesses a relatively long half-life of 20 - 21 days. The normal range of albumin is 35-45g/l, the values giving evidence of significant malnutrition in seniors lie below 28g/l [54, 70]. Albumin decreased below 35g/l does not have to be associated with malnutrition according to Kuzuya et al. [46]. In seniors with a normal test of ordinary activities of ADL (19-20) and medium decreased ADL (2-18), correction between the levels of serum albumin and other nutritional markers was demonstrated, whereas in patients with a significant decrease in ADL (0-1), a decrease in albumin below 35g/l was not demonstrated as a suitable indicator of malnutrition and led to its overestimation. This, however, does not hold true for the shift of evaluation of albumin below 28g/l. Albumin concentration may be influenced by the state of hydration, shifts between the intravascular and extracellular spaces, and liver or renal diseases. It is also a negative acute phase protein and it is necessary to relate its values to the values of CRP [27, 42, 54]. A significant negative correlation between albumin and CRP in patients of higher age is shown in the study of Ravaglia et al. [66].

Prealbumin

The role of prealbumin is particularly the transfer of thyroxin and collaboration in the transport of retinol-binding protein (RBP), with which it forms a complex in the ratio 1:1. It contains also a high concentration of tryptophan, which significantly participates in proteosynthesis. Of all serum proteins, prealbumin possesses the shortest biological half-life of 1 – 2 days; therefore it is most suitable for the evaluation of acute protein malnutrition and immediate success of possible nutritional therapy in the initial stages of realimentation. Prealbumin is capable to capture part of patients already at risk of malnutrition because at least 44% of patients with decreased prealbumin still have normal values of albumin [87]. At present it is an advantageous marker as well as for monitoring the nutritional state, when the trend of its development is more important than the absolute values. The normal values of prealbumin are 0.2-0.4g/l, within a range of 0.10-0.20g/l it is a mild degree of malnutrition, and serious malnutrition is signaled by the values below 0.10g/l [54]. But it also belongs to the negative acute phase proteins (its synthesis is suppressed by anti-inflammatory cytokines) and it is necessary to evaluate it in relation with CRP [27, 31, 53, 71]. Lower values may occur also in the affections of liver functions (hepatitides, liver cirrhosis) and zinc deficit [42, 67].

Transferin

Transferin is the principal transport protein for iron in plasma. It is a beta-globulin synthesized mainly in the liver, in a small amount also in the reticuloendothelial system, testes and ovaries. The half-life of transferin is 5 – 7 days, and it is an early marker of protein malnutrition, but it is less reliable, having lower specificity and sensitivity. On the other hand, an increase in the transferin level sensitively indicates the onset of a positive nitrogen balance. The physiological range of transferin is 2-3.6g/l, the serum concentration giving evidence of malnutrition is below 1.5g/l [27, 54], but it may be significantly influenced by the amount of iron in the organism, an acute inflammatory disease (negative acute phase protein), malignity in progress, a surgery or chronic hepatopathy [53]. When evaluating transferin, it is suitable to know the state of iron metabolism, C-reactive protein and the proteosynthetic liver function. In patients with malnutrition and concurrent sideropenic anemia it is unsuitable as a single marker [42, 87].

Cholinesterase

Cholinesterase is an enzyme produced by hepatocytes and secreted to blood plasma. It influences the neuromuscular junction of skeletal bones. The normal range is 88-215 μkat/l. The half-life of cholinesterase is 5 – 7 days, its level correlates well with the albumin level [54]. Due to its relatively short half-life and low price, cholinesterase can be employed to monitor the nutritional state. A decrease in cholinesterase can be demonstrated in malnutrition (the risk level is that below 88 μkat/l), but also in hypercatabolic states in severe infections and its level is dependent on the function of the liver and on some medicaments (physostigmine, cyclophosphamide, lithium etc.). A decrease in cholesterol level is usually significant in the affection of the hepatic parenchyma most frequently in chronic diseases of the liver due to inhibition of the synthesis and number of producing cells. In more severe affections of the liver, it is not possible to take into account the values of cholinesterase in nutritional evaluation, because a low level rather than the state of nutrition reflects a deficit of liver proteosynthesis [27, 42, 87].

Serum Lipids

Bioindicators of malnutrition are some parameters of lipid metabolism. A decrease in total cholesterol, LDL and HDL indicates an energetic deficit and specific manifestations of malnutrition. Though it is generally accepted that in serious malnutrition cholesterolemia is decreased (manifestations of an energetic deficit, worse availability of acetyl-coenzyme-A), it does not generally hold true. In severely cachectic individuals with mental anorexia, cholesterolemia is often increased up to grossly pathological values. It can be explained by stimulation of the synthesis of cholesterol in deprivation of the absorption of cholesterol from the gastrointestinal tract. Interpretation of plasma concentrations of triacylglycerols in malnutrition is even less unambiguous. This parameter reflects rather the topical state of the intake of nutrients than long-term consequences of malnutrition [27, 35, 87].

The study by Blaha et al. [5, 76] demonstrated a significantly lower serum concentration of cholesterol ($p<0.05$), HDL cholesterol and TAG in longeval out-patients (over 90 years) versus the control group (under 89 years).

Total Cholesterol

The level of total cholesterol is a relatively sensitive marker of energy malnutrition and correlates better with the body-mass index than the level of albumin. At the same time, however, the levels of total cholesterol and albumin do not have to correlate with each other. The normal range is 2.2-5.2mmol/l, the levels below 2.0mmol/l indicate, after the exclusion of the influencing factors, long-term energetic insufficiency [27, 54]. For evaluation of cholesterol it is necessary to know at the same time the values of thyreoideal enzymes, liver functions and the concurrently administered medication (hypolipidemics) [87].

C-Reactive Protein (CRP)

CRP is the dominant acute phase protein. It ranks among pentraxins – a group of proteins occurring in all vertebrates and ensuring defence of the organism. CRP activates the complement system by both the classic and alternative way, and by binding to various ligands (proteins from disintegrated cells, polysaccharide envelope of pneumococci C, etc.) it protects the organism from the action of necrotic products from disintegrated cells (16). Another capacity of CRP is regulation of acute inflammatory processes by influencing thrombocytes by the effect on the metabolism of prostaglandins and also hindrance of stimulation of T-lymphocytes and release of lymphokines. It also acts on phagocytosis by influencing granulocytic and monocytic macrophages. An important task of CRP is also opsonization and rapid removal of fragments of nucleic acids and histones, which prevents the development of autoantibodies against these elements [24, 27, 53, 66].

CRP is produced by the liver and after stimulation there is an increase after 6-8 hours and the maximal values are achieved in 24-48 hours. The normal range is 0-5 mg/l. Elevation of CRP values is accompanied by acute inflammatory diseases, in the case of malignant diseases and the majority of rheumatic diseases the increase is smaller. It is important to continuously monitor the serum level in the course of therapy, which correlates with the activity of the disease (5, 21). After successful treatment with antibiotics there is a rapid decrease in CRP, in the case of unsuccessful treatment the increased level persists or it may even rise. Viral infection, in contrast to a bacterial one, is not usually accompanied by an increase in CRP [27, 54].

Hematological and Immunological Examinations

The hematological and immunological examinations include particularly the determination of the absolute number of lymphocytes; malnutrition may be indicated by anemia (due to deficiency of iron, folic acid or vitamin B12). In the elderly, there is often an anergic reaction to immunological intradermal skin tests [86]. The monitoring of neopterin in urine is also advisable. To evaluate the state of immunity in connection with the state of nutrition, it is possible to employ special immunological examinations such as the determination of the level of immunoglobulins and the examination of the subpopulations of CD4, CD8 lymphocytes (at present rather as part of research tasks, in common clinical practice these examinations are not routinely used) [45, 63].

Absolute Number of Lymphocytes

Malnutrition results in a decrease in the function of the immunity system first at the level of cellular and subsequently also humoral immunity. The absolute number of lymphocytes is evaluated, whose normal value should not decrease below 1 500/μl; below this limit the risk of malnutrition is increased and a decrease below 900/μl means a significant affection of immunity with a high risk of severe malnutrition [53, 87]. It is necessary to first exclude other etiology of decreased lymphocytes (hemato-oncological diseases, TBC, viroses etc.). According to Pirlich [65] and Omran [63], a decrease in the absolute number of lymphocytes can be used as a marker of malnutrition in elderly patients; on the other hand, Kuzuya [47] doubts it.

4. Functional Examination – Dynamometry

Judgement of function condition of the muscle tissue is necessary for judging the seriousness of a clinical state. For outpatient monitoring hand dynamometer is suitable, which measures the strength of muscle grip (hand grip) [30]. In the case of a nutrition disorder, muscle strength is usually decreased. Muscle strength decreases physiologically in the old age, but in malnourished seniors the decrease is more significant. A disadvantage of dynamometry is that especially in the old age it could be considerably influenced by the non-cooperation of the patient or his disability to grip the dynamometer due to rheumatic diseases of hand joints [16, 87].

Prevention of Malnutrition in the Elderly

As follows from the title, malnutrition is in fact insufficient nutrition. A preventive measure is thus in any case a balanced, varied and energy-sufficient diet, which fulfils the rules of rational nutrition and at the same time its form is suitable for seniors. Furthermore, it is necessary to avoid, if possible, all risk factors of malnutrition in the elderly (see Table 1).

THERAPY OF MALNUTRITION AND DEFICIENCY STATES IN THE ELDERLY

1. Dietary Measures and Adjustment of Dietary Habits

With advancing age the consequences of incorrect dietary habits are summed up and the will and capability to change them is decreased [55]. This is also the reason why certain adjustments of dietary habits are necessary in nearly all seniors. In the case of the patients who already suffer from malnutrition or are at risk of it, cooperation with a dietologist and specific recommendations made-to-measure for the patient are advisable even before cachexia develops [12]. In two thirds of patients it is enough to maintain a satisfactory state of nutrition [51, 59].

In higher age, peroral nutrition is unambiguously the method of choice. Healthy nutrition must be sufficient regarding energy and with a balanced content of sugars, fats and proteins. At the same time it must contain a sufficient amount of vitamins, trace elements, roughage and liquids. The optimal ratio of the individual components of food should be 10-15% of proteins, 55-75% of sugars and up to 30% of fats [87]. The intake of crude roughage should reach 20-25g a day, in cholesterol it is up to 300mg a day, the intake of fruit and vegetables should be higher than 400g and salts up to 6g. In the elderly there occurs an increased action of free radicals and an increase in diseases resulting from it. An increased supply of antioxidants in the diet can partially suppress their unwanted influence. In the diet it is necessary to take into account a gradual transition from solid foods via the mash diet to the liquid one, omission of less well absorbed dishes, transition to softer foodstuffs and bouillons. Proteins in food can be obtained, besides meat, in another source such as, e.g. cottage cheese, cheese, yogurts, milk (acidophilus milk or buttermilk are better) or eggs [12]. Appetite can be positively affected even by a small volume of beer, and if the patient asks for it, there is no reason to refuse his request.

In the selection of food it is always necessary to take into account the individual wishes of the patient, his or her taste preferences and dietary habits. Besides the nutrition values the appearance of offered food is also important because the patient should have appetite and enjoy the meal. Food should be varied, arranged in an appetizing way and of various colours. Smaller meals served more frequently are more suitable, they should be eaten slowly, and the patient should not hurry. The patient should eat in a well ventilated room because unpleasant smell decreases appetite. Increased oral intake is substantially supported by adjusted medication and discontinuation of administration of all dispensable medicaments as well as active treatment of pain, constipation, possible affection in the oral cavity, nausea, and depression [65].

2. Enteral Nutrition

If it is at all possible, enteral nutrition is always preferred to parenteral one, and the intake per os prior to nutrition administered via a tube. Enteral nutrition is more physiological due to the incorporation of the function of the gastrointestinal tract and improvement of immunity response [2, 7, 57].

Sipping

If we are not able to ensure a satisfactory peroral intake only by adjusting the dietary habits and the patient is able to receive food only per os, nutritional additions in the form of drinking between meals are suitable. At present both complete formulae, as well as preparations containing individual components of nutrition are available. It is also possible to individually select various flavours or special compositions suitable, e.g. for diabetic patients or patients with defects [87]. Sipping is better tolerated if it is administered cooled.

Tube Nutrition and Percutaneous Gastrostomy (PEG)

An introduction of a thin nasogastric or nasojejunal tube and administration of nutrition via a tube is simple, cheap, and sufficient to ensure additional energy intake for several weeks. At the same time there is a certain impairment of the comfort of the patient, some patients bear tubes badly and their introduction, in spite of its thin diameter, is frequently stressing for the patient [7, 52]. Percutaneous gastrostomy (PEG) is not introduced if the expected period of survival of the patient is longer than 3 months (in individual cases shorter) and a long-term necessity of enteral nutrition administration is assumed. Excepting the act of introduction, PEG is relatively better tolerated than a tube. In both cases, however, there is a risk of aspiration and subsequent pulmonary complications (due to deterioration of withdrawal reflexes), which is smaller when the tube is administered as far as the proximal jejunum. The nasogastric tube can be used only to administer mixed home food or mass-produced bolus nutrition manufactured by a firm, administration of nutrition into the jejunum is usually continuous via a nutritional pump and only sterile proprietary preparations can be used [38].

There are several types of enteral nutrition. Polymeric enteral nutritions are lactose-free, cholesterol-free, they do not contain gluten and resorbable remains. The source of nitrogen is purified protein, e.g. albumin, caseinate, egg albumin. They are very well resorbable in the gastrointestinal tract, but it is necessary to maintain a sufficient resorption area – at least 60cm of the jejunum. Oligopeptidic enteral nutrition is used in patients with an increased consumption of nitrogen (patients in serious catabolism) and in deteriorated absorption capability of the digestive tract. Nitrogen is here replaced by protein hydrolysates containing medium- and low-molecular peptides, saccharides are represented by low-molecular dextrins, lipids, mostly from dyer's saffron containing MCT. Organ-specific enteral nutritions are_highly special nutritional preparations making use of the fact that some nutritional substrates in pharmacological doses act favourably in the treatment of some pathological conditions [72, 87].

3. Parenteral Nutrition

Parenteral nutrition is used in the case of contraindication of enteral nutrition in the affections of the gastrointestinal tract or malabsorption. According to the type and degree of malnutrition and the degree of affection of the gastrointestinal tract it is possible to choose from several types of parenteral nutrition.

The supplementary parenteral nutrition does not cover the whole day requirements of the patient in all nutritional components. Full (total) parenteral nutrition is the main source of energy, supplementing all necessary components including vitamins and trace elements even in the long term. Special organ-specific nutrition includes, besides the principal energy and nutritional substrates also specific nutritional substrates with pharmacological effects (glutamine, ω-3 fatty acids, and others.) [72].

If we expect a shorter period of administration of parenteral nutrition (a maximum of 2-3 weeks), nutrition can be administered into the peripheral vein. Another indication for peripheral parenteral nutrition is the case when cannulation of the central vein is not possible or contraindicated. For a transient period of time, peripheral parenteral nutrition can be administered even in the case of catheter sepsis or bacteraemia caused by a central venous catheter, if nutrition must continue. The periphery can be supplied only with supplementary parenteral nutrition with low osmolality (less than 1200mosmol/kg). An advantage of peripheral parenteral nutrition is an easy access to the venous system, a fewer number of complications and their easy recognition.

If long-term parenteral nutrition is necessary, a catheter is introduced to the central vein (vena subclavia, vena jugularis). Via the central vein it is possible to administer both supplementary and total parenteral nutrition and solutions with increased osmolality. A risk of the administration of total parenteral nutrition is intestinal atrophy, attenuation of the intestinal immunity barrier and an increased risk of infectious complications by the penetration of the microorganisms substances that are normally found in the body from the lumen through the intestinal wall or also by catheter sepsis when a central venous catheter is introduced.

At present the most frequently employed form of parenteral nutrition is the use of all-in-one sacs, either mass-produced by a firm, or prepared directly on the spot [87].

REFERENCES

[1] Aronow, W.S., Fleg, J.L. *Cardiovascular Disease in the Elderly*. Marcel Dekker; 2004.

[2] Bankhead, R., Boullata, J.I., Compher, CH.W. Clinical Nutrition. *Enteral and Tube Feeding*. Philadelphia: Elsevier Saunders; 2005.

[3] Bauer, J.M., Volkert, D., Wirth, R., Vellas, B., Thomas, D., Kondrup, J. et al. Diagnosing malnutrition in the elderly. *Dtsch. Med. Wochenschr.* 2006; 131 (5): 223-227.

[4] Beneš, P. Základy umělé výživy. *Nutriční péče pro nemocniční praxi.* Praha: Maxdorf Jessenius; 1999.

[5] Bláha, V., Zadák, Z. Nutriční stav nemocných v pokročilém věku a u dlouhověkých. *Geriatria* 1995; 1: 25-28.

[6] Caballero, B., Allen, L., Prentice, A. *Encyclopedia of Human Nutrition.* Oxford: Elsevier Academic Press; 2005.

[7] Casarett, D., Kapo, J., Caplan, A. Appropriate Use of Artificial Nutrition and Hydratation - Fundamental Principles and Recommendations. *N. Eng. J. Med.* 2005; 353 (24): 2607-2612.

[8] Carmeli, E., Coleman, R., Reznick, A.Z. The biochemistry of aging muscle. *Exp. Geront.* 2002; 37: 477-489.

[9] Cederholm, T., Jägrén, C., Hellström, K. Outcome of Protein-Energy Malnutrition in Elderly Medical Patients. *Am. J. Med.* 1995; 98: 67-74.

[10] Corish, C.A., Kennedy, N.P. Protein-energy undernutrition in hospital in-patients. *Br. J. Nutr.* 2000; 83: 575-591.

[11] Devoto, G., Gallo, F., Marchello, C., Racchi, O., Garbarini, R., Bonassi, S. et al. Prealbumin serum levels as a useful tool in the assessment of malnutrition in hospitalized patients. *Clin. Chem.* 2006; 52: 2281-5.

[12] Doberský, P., Šimončič, R., Bučko, A. a kol. Dietní systém pro nemocnice. *Osveta*, 1983.

[13] Doherty, T.J. Invited review: Aging and sarcopenia. *J. Appl. Physiol.* 2003; 95 (4): 717-1727.

[14] Dorrens, J., Rennie, M.J. Effects of ageing and human whole body and muscle protein turnover. *Scand. J. Med. Sci. Sports* 2003; 13 (1): 26-33.

[15] Duerksen, D.R., Yeo, T.A., Siemens, J.L., O'Conno, M.P. The validity and eproducibility of clinical assessment of nutritional status in the elderly. *Nutr.* 2000; 16 (9): 740-744.

[16] Ferrucci, L., Penninx, B.W., Volpato, S., Harris, T.B., Bandeen-Roche, K., Balfour, J. et al. Change in muscle strength explains accelerated decline of physical function in older women with high interleukin-6 serum levels. *J. Am. Geriatr. Soc.* 2002; 50 (12): 1947-1954.

[17] Fidanza, F. Nutritional Status Assessment. *A manual for population studies*. London: Chapman and Hall; 1991.

[18] Fuhrman, M.P., Charney, P., Mueller, C.M. Hepatic proteins and nutrition assessment. *J. Am. Diet Assoc.* 2004; 104: 1258-64.

[19] Fulle, S., Protasi, F., Di Tano, G., Pietrangelo, T., Beltramin, A., Boncompagni, S. et al. The contribution of reactive oxygen species to sarcopenia and muscle ageing. *Exp. Geront.* 2004; 39: 17-19.

[20] Gaillard, C., Alix, E., Sallé, A., Berrut, G., Ritz, P. Energy requirements in frail elderly people: A review of the literature. *Clin. Nutr.* 2007; 26: 16-24.

[21] Giovannini, I., Chiarla, C., Giuliante, F., Vellone, M., Zadak, Z., Nuzzo, G. Hypocholesterolemia in Surgical Trauma, Sepsis, other Acute Conditions and Critical Illness. In: Kramer, M.A., editor: *Trends in Cholesterol Research.* New York: Nova Science Publishers; 2005, 137-161.

[22] Greenlund, L.J., Nair, K.S. Sarcopenia - consequences, mechanisms, and potential therapies. *Mech. Ageing. Dev.* 2003; 124(3): 287-299.

[23] Guigoz, Y., Vellas, B., Garry, P.J. Mini Nutritional Assessment: A practical assessment tool for grading the nutritional state of elderly patients. In: Vellas, B., Guigoz, Y., Garry, P.J. et al. The Mini Nutritional Assessment: MNA. Nutrition in the Elderly. *Facts and Research in Gerontology*. Supplement 2. New York: Springe Publishing Co; 1994: 15-59.

[24] Harris, T.B., Ferrucci, L., Tracy, R.P., Corti, M.C., Wacholder, S., Ettinger, W.H. et al. Associations of elevated Interleukin-6 and C-Reactive protein levels with mortality in the elderly. *Am. J. Med.* 1999; 106: 506-512.

[25] Hazzard, W.R., Blass, J.P., Halter, J.P., Ouslander, J.G., Tinetti, M.E. *Principles of Geriatric Medicine and Gerontology*. McGraw-Hill Companies; 2003.

[26] Holmerová, I., Jurašková, B., Zikmundová, K. *Vybrané kapitoly z gerontologie.* Praha: Česká alzheimerovská společnost; 2003.

[27] Hrnciarikova, D., Zadak, Z., Juraskova, B., Hyspler, R., Klemera, P. Bioindicators of malnutrition and inflammation in the elderly. In: Bernhardt, N.E., Kasko, A.M. editors. *Nutrition for Middle Aged and Elderly.* New York: Nova Publishers, 2008: 371-387.

[28] Hronek, M. *Výživa ženy v obdobích těhotenství a kojení.* Praha: Maxdorf Jessenius; 2004.

[29] Ingenbleek, Y., Young, V.R. Significance of prealbumin in protein metabolism. *Clin. Chem. Lab. Med.* 2002; 40: 1281-91.

[30] Janda, V. a kol. *Svalové funkční testy.* Praha: GRADA Publishing; 2004.

[31] Johnson, A.M., Merlini, G., Sheldon, J., Ichihara, K. Clinical indications for plasma protein assays: transthyretin (prealbumin) in inflammation and malnutrition. *Clin. Chem. Lab. Med.* 2007; 45 (3): 419-426.

[32] Junquiera, J.C., Soares, E.C., Filho, H.R.C., Hoehr, N.F., Magro, D.O., Ueno, M. Nutritional Risk Factors for Postoperative Complications in Brazilian Elderly Patients Undergoing Major Elective Surgery. *Nutr.* 2003; 19: 321-326.

[33] Jurašková, B. Nutriční podpora v geriatrii. *Lékařské listy* 2006; 13: 10-13.

[34] Jurašková, B., Hrnčiariková, D., Holmerová, I., Kalvach, Z. Poruchy výživy ve stáří. *Medicína pro praxi* 2007; 9(4): 443-446.

[35] Jurašková, B. Význam monitorování antioxidační kapacity a metabolismu lipidů v procesu stárnutí. Čes ger rev 2006; 4 (2): 72-76.

[36] Jurašková, B., Zadák, Z. Poruchy výživy ve stáří. *Zdravotnické noviny (příl. Lékařské listy)* 2002; 51 (51/52): 11-12.

[37] Kagansky, N., Berner, Y., Koren-Morag, N., Perelman, L., Knobler, H., Levy, S. Poor nutritional habits are predictors of poor outcome in very old hospitalized patiens. *Am. J. Clin. Nutr.* 2005; 82 (4): 784-791.

[38] Kalvach, Z., Zadák, Z., Jirák, R., Zavázalová, H., Sucharda, P. *Geriatrie a gerontologie*. Praha: Grada Publishing; 2004.

[39] Kalvach, Z. a kol. *Úvod do gerontologie a geriatrie*. Praha: Karolinum; 1997.

[40] Kalvach, Z. a kol. *Vybrané kapitoly z geriatrie a medicíny chronických stavů.* Praha: Karolinum; 1995.

[41] Kamel, H.K. Sarcopenia and aging. *Nutr. Rev*. 2003; 61: 157-167.

[42] Kohout, P. *Dokumentace a hodnocení nutričního stavu pacientů*. Praha: Maxdorf; 2004.

[43] Kohout, P. *Výživa u pacientů s idiopatickými střevními záněty*. Praha: Maxdorf Jessenius; 2004.

[44] Kondrup, J., Johansen, N., Plum, L.M., Bak, L., Højlund Larsen, I., Martinsen, A. et al. Incidence of nutritional risk and causes of inadequate nutritional care in hospitals. *Clin. Nutr*. 2002; 21 (6): 461-468.

[45] Kopecký, O. et al. *Laboratorní vyšetření v klinické imunologii a alergologii.* Hradec Králové: GARAMON; 2004.

[46] Kuzuya, M., Izawa, S., Enoki, H., Okada, K., Iguchi, A. Is serum albumin a good marker for malnutrition in the physically impaired elderly? *Clin. Nutr.* 2007; 26: 84-90.

[47] Kuzuya, M., Kanda, S., Koike, T., Suzuki, Y., Iguchi, A. Lack of correlation between total lymphocyte count and nutritional status in the elderly. *Clin. Nutr.* 2005; 24: 427-432.

[48] Kyle, U.G., Genton, L., Pichard, C. Hospital length of stay and nutritional status. *Curr. Opin. Clin Nutr. Metab. Care* 2005; 8 (4): 397-402.

[49] Kyle, U.G., Unger, P., Mensi, N., Genton, L., Pichard, C. Nutrition Status in Patients Younger and Older Than 60 y at Hospital Admission: A Controlled Population Study in 995 Subjects. *Nutr.* 2002; 18: 463-469.

[50] Kyle, U.G., Pirlich, M., Scuetz, T., Luebke, H.J., Lochs, H., Pichard, C. Prevalence of malnutrition in 1760 patients at hospital admission: a controlled population study of body composition. *Clin. Nutr*. 2003; 22: 473-481.

[51] Lasheras, C., González, C., García, A., Patterson, A.M., Fernández, S. Dietary intake and biochemical indicators of nutritional status in an elderly institutionalized and non-institutionalized population. *Nutr. Res.* 1999; 19 (9): 1299-1312.

[52] MacFie, J. Ethics of artificial nutrition. *Nutr*. 2006; 34 (12): 548-550.

[53] Macallan, D. Malnutrition and infection. *Medicine* 2005; 33: 14-16.

[54] Masopust, J. *Klinická biochemie – požadování a hodnocení biochemických vyšetření.* Praha: Karolinum; 1998.

[55] Michalko, L., Michalík, D. Vybrané parametre výživy a stravovacie zvyky u osôb vyšších vekových skupín. *Čes a Slov Gastroent* 1999; 53 (1): 3-8.

[56] Morley, J.E. Anorexia, Sarcopenia, and Aging. *Nutr*. 2001; 17: 660-663.

[57] Morley, J.E. Symposium on „Nutrition and the elderly". Protein-energy malnutrition in older subjects. *Proc. Nutr. Soc.* 1998; 57: 587-592.

[58] Morrison, G., Hark, L. Medical Nutrition and Disease. *Blackwell Science;* 1996.

[59] Musil, D. Poruchy výživy a využití nutriční podpory u starších lidí a u chronicky nemocných. *Praktický lékař* 2001; 81 (9): 516-520.

[60] Mühlberg, W., Weidermann, G., Stedtfeld, H.W., Sieber, C. Low Total Protein Increases Injury Risk in the Elderly. *J. Am. Ger. Soc.* 2004; 52 (2): 324-325.

[61] Navrátilová, M., Češková, E., Sobotka, L. *Klinická výživa v psychiatrii.* Praha: Maxdorf Jessenius; 2000.

[62] Norman, K., Pichard, C., Lochs, H., Pirlich, M. Prognostic impact of disease-related malnutrition. *Clin. Nutr*. 2008; 27: 5-15.

[63] Omran, M.L., Morley, J.E. Assessment of protein energy malnutrition in older persons, Part II: laboratory evaluation. *Nutrition* 2000; 16: 131-40.

[64] Pedersen, M., Bruunsgaard, H., Weis, N., Hendel, H.W., Andreassen, B.U., Eldrup, E. et al. Circulating levels of TNF-alpha and IL-6-relation to truncal fat mass and muscle mass in healthy elderly individuals and in patients with type-2 diabetes. *Mech. Ageing Dev*. 2003; 124(4): 495-502.

[65] Pirlich, M., Lochs, H. Nutrition in the elderly. *Best Pract. Res. Clin. Gastroenter.* 2001; 15: 869-884.

[66] Ravaglia, G., Forti, P., Maioli, F., Brunetti, N., Martelli, M., Talerico, T. et al. Peripheral blood markers of inflammation and functional impairment in elderly community-dwellers. *Exp. Geront*. 2004; 39: 1415-1422.

[67] Robinson, M.K., Trujillo, E.B., Mogensen, K.M., Rounds, J., McManus, K., Jacobs, D.O. Improving nutritional screening of hospitalized

patients: the role of prealbumin. *J. Parenter. Enteral. Nutr.* 2003; 27: 389-95.

[68] Roubenoff, R. Catabolism of aging: is it an inflammatory process? *Curr. Opin. Clin. Nutr. Metab. Care* 2003; 6 (3): 295-299.

[69] Ruiz-Lopez, M.D., Artacho, R., Oliva, P., Moreno-Torres, R., Bolanos, J., de Teresa, C. et al. Nutritional risk in institutionalized older women determined by the Mini Nutritional Assessment test. What are the main factors? *Nutr.* 2003; 19 (9): 767-71.

[70] Seiler, W.O. Clinical pictures of malnutrition in ill elderly subjects. *Nutrition* 2001; 17: 496-8.

[71] Shenkin, A. Serum Prealbumin: Is It a Marker of Nutritional Status or of Risk of Malnutrition? *Clin. Chem.* 2006; 52 (12): 2177-79.

[72] Shikora, S.A., Blackburn, G.L. Nutrition support. *Theory and Therapeutics.* Chapman and Hall; 1996

[73] Sobotka, L. *Basics in Clinical Nutrition.* Praha: Galén; 2004.

[74] Solichová, D., Jurašková, B., Brátová, M. Lipid profile, antioxidants and longevity. *Nutr.* 2000; 16 (11/12): 1129.

[75] Solichová, D., Melichar, B., Bláha, V., Brátová, M., Jurašková, B., Zadák, Z. Biochemical monitoring in gerontology. *Acta Medica* 1999; 42 (2): 5.

[76] Solichova, D., Melichar, B., Blaha, V., Klejna, M., Vavrova, J., Palicka, V., Zadak, Z. Biochemical profile and survival in nonagerians. *Clin. Bioch.* 2001; 34 (7): 563-569.

[77] Solichová, D., Melichar, B., Klejna, M., Jurašková, B., Bláha, V., Žďánský, P., Zadák, Z. Stanovení neopterinu v moči u gerontologických pacientů. *Čes ger. Rev.* 2003; 1 (3), 32- 38.

[78] Sullivan, D.H., Sun, S., Walls, R.C. Protein-Energy Undernutrition Among Elderly Hospitalized Patients. *JAMA* 1999; 281: 2013-2019.

[79] Sungurtekin, H., Sungurtekin, U., Hanci, V., Erdem, E. Comparison of Two Nutrition Assessment Techniques in Hospitalized Patients. *Nutrition* 2004; 20: 428-432.

[80] Topinková, E., Neuwirth, J. *Geriatrie pro praktického lékaře.* Praha: GRADA Publishing; 1995.

[81] Topinková, E. *Geriatrie pro praxi.* Praha: Galén; 2005.

[82] Topinková, E. Jak správně a včas diagnostikovat demenci. *Manuál pro klinickou praxi.* Praha: UCB Pharma; 1999.

[83] Topinková, E. Využití standardizovaných škál pro hodnocení stavu výživy u starších nemocných. *Čes. Ger. Rev.* 2003; 1 (1): 6-11.

[84] Vellas, B., Guigoz, Y., Baumgartner, M., Garry, P.J., Lauque, S., Albarede, J.L. Relationships between nutritional markers and the mini-nutritional assessement in older persons. *J. Am. Geriatr. Soc.* 2000; 48 (10): 1300-9.

[85] Zadák, Z. Vitaminy a mikroelementy ve stáří. *Čes. Ger. Rev.* 2003; 1 (1): 12-16.

[86] Zadák, Z. a kol. *Vybrané kapitoly z metabolismu a klinické výživy.* Praha: Karolinum; 1997.

[87] Zadák, Z. *Výživa v intenzivní péči*. Praha: GRADA Publishing, 2002.

In: Malnutrition: Risk Factors ...
Editor: J.B. Knudsen

ISBN: 978-1-62100-351-9

Chapter 3

MALNUTRITION IN INFLAMMATORY BOWEL DISEASES: CROHN'S DISEASE AND ULCERATIVE COLITIS

Hatzitolios Apostolos[1] and Tsiaousi Eleni[2]
[1]Aristotle University of Thessaloniki, 1st Medical Propedeutic Department, Ahepa University Hospital, Thessaloniki, Greece
[2]Aristotle University of Thessaloniki, 2nd Medical Department, Ippokration Hospital, Thessaloniki, Greece

ABSTRACT

Malnutrition is diagnosed in 80% of hospitalized Crohn's disease patients and in 20-40% of outpatients with Crohn's disease, whereas ulcerative colitis patients usually avoid the severe complication of malnutrition because in most of the cases the small intestine is spared. Nevertheless, malnutrition can become prevalent in periods of severe clinical relapse even in ulcerative colitis patients. Several factors contribute to the emergence of malnutrition in inflammatory bowel diseases, with the inflammatory activity, duration of the illness or flares of the disease, the extent of the inflamed intestine and the function of the intestinal epithelium being the most important. Decreased food intake, macro- and micronutrient malabsorption and increased intestinal nutrient loss lead to a state of nutrient deficiency and body weight loss.

Oral or enteral nutrition is by far recommended in terms of improvement of bowel function and nutritional status. Parenteral nutrition is indicated only in cases of toxic megacolon, ileus or partial ileus, severe malabsorption syndrome, such as short bowel syndrome and growth retardation in children and adolescents for the acute phase when oral or enteral nutrition is not possible, since parenteral nutrition per se does not lead to sustained clinical remission, fistulae healing or avoidance of surgery.

INTRODUCTION

Nutritional status plays a crucial role in several debilitating diseases with chronic and relapsing course such as inflammatory bowel diseases. Low Body Mass Index (BMI), malnutrition and specific nutrient deficiencies are frequently encountered by physicians in their management of IBD patients. Since 25% of them represent the pediatric population of IBD, growth retardation is a major clinical issue that has to be dealed with or in ideal circumstances prevented.

The pathophysiology of undernutrition is multifactorial and complex and therefore a thorough nutritional assessment is required before measures are taken. It has been established that malnutrition can have an adverse impact in several gastrointestinal diseases with direct negative effect in quality of life, disease course, in disease free survival and in some fortunately rare cases in survival in total. Although Crohn's disease and Ulcerative colitis share common disease pathways and project a sometimes similar clinical expression they differ significantly as far as the nutritional status is concerned. Crohn's disease patients may present underweight or malnourished in particular during severe disease flares, whereas patients with Ulcerative colitis rarely present with significant nutritional deficits. Nevertheless in periods of active disease it is not odd to find malnourished UC patients and therefore clinical awareness should rise to maximum.

Specific dietary programs with multiple do's and don'ts, enteral and parenteral, supplementary or exclusive nutrition have been suggested and tried in clinical trials with primary endpoint the correction of nutritional deficit. However the primary goal may sometimes differ in certain groups of patients. Enteral nutritional supplementation has been given as primary therapy especially for pediatric CD for induction of remission. Alternative to maintenance pharmacotherapy in CD or supplementary, EN has been tried with conflicting results. Parenteral nutrition is inappropriate and should be reserved for patients with ileus or subileus of the small intestine, intestinal fistulae, major gastrointestinal infections, small bowel syndrome and severe and life-threatening malnourishment, in short courses followed promptly by enteral and/or oral nutrition.

For UC enteral nutrition, parenteral nutrition and specific diet restrictions are inappropriate according to the guidelines of European Crohn's and Colitis Organization.

PATHOPHYSIOLOGY AND PREVALENCE OF MALNUTRITION IN IBD

An estimated 70-80% of hospitalized patients with inflammatory bowel diseases and 20-40% of outpatients with Crohn's disease present with evident signs of malnutrition or nutritional deficits (Van Patter 1954, Lanfranchi 1984). Geerling et al report a lower body weight and BMI among recently diagnosed patients with CD or UC in comparison with age and sex matched controls which gives emphasis to the fact that impairment of nutrition may present early in the course of the disease or at presentation (Geerling 2000). However during disease flares malnutrition may become prevalent even if the patient is adequately nourished or even overweight. Mijac et al in an attempt to assess the prevalence of undernutrition among 23 patients with active Crohn's disease, 53 patients with active UC and 30 controls found that the prevalence of undernutrition and severe undernutrition among patients with active IBD was 25-69,7% and 1,3-31,6% respectively according to the implemented method of assessment. On the contrary CD patients in remission were better nourished with 38,9% of them being reported as malnourished (Mijac 2010).

The pathophysiology of malnutrition in IBD is usually multifactorial with several mechanisms being responsible for lower nutrient intake or high nutrient loss, which often intertwine and may lead to severe body weight loss or micro- and macronutrient deficits. One of the main causes of lower food ingestion is anorexia (Hartman 2009). Increased levels of pro-inflammatory cytokines such as Tumor Necrosis factor-a and interleukins 1,6,17,23 which in combination with alterations in the secretion of serotonin by the hypothalamus are responsible for the emergence of anorexia (Murch 1998, Ballinger 2000). These cytokines are often responsible for the hypermetabolic state which is encountered in several chronic diseases. The increased Resting Energy Expenditure of IBD patients during active disease periods may lead to gradual body weight loss if the new energy requirements are not met (Zoli 1996).

Apart from this, fear of food ingestion due to abdominal pain, nausea, vomiting and disturbing diarrhea is a serious complication of the disease process since the amount of food ingested is significantly smaller. Another important issue to keep in mind is the restrictions in diet which are quite often imposed by physicians to IBD patients in an attempt to prevent disease flares or severe diarrhoic or abdominal pain episodes. In certain circumstances it is very difficult for patients to maintain proper body weight since a great number of food types is forbidden for them sometimes in an exaggerating manner. Patients tend for example to avoid certain food types such as dairies, which are considered to contribute to disease flares, receiving as a consequence inadequate amount of calcium (Jowett 2004).

Nevertheless sometimes even if the patients follow a more rich in nutrients diet with proper amount of caloric intake this may not be enough for them to avoid malnutrition. Active inflammation with infiltration of the intestinal mucosa and submucosa in UC and all intestinal layers in CD of mononuclear cells and polymorphonuclear neutrophil cells which produce pro-inflammatory mediators may lead to extensive loss of the intestinal absorptive surface. Furthermore malnutrition may be attributed to several iatrogenic interventions: surgical and pharmaceutical. Extensive surgical intestinal resections or intestinal bypasses and fistulae are often responsible for the diminished absorption of nutrients. Small bowel syndrome after major resections or severe fistulizing and stricturing disease activity may contribute to severe or even life threatening malnutrition.

Table 1. Pathophysiology of malnutritionHypermetabolic state Poor nutrient intake Intestinal loss Malabsorption

Increased resting energy expenditure (REE)	Loss of appetite (TNF driven?)	Diarrhea (fluid, electrolyte and nutrient loss)	Deceased intestinal epithelium
Gastrointestinal and general infections	Abdominal pain, nausea, bloating, vomiting, diarrhea	Vomiting	Surgical bypass, fistulae
Elevated pro-inflammatory and anti-inflammatory cytokines	Diet restrictions (sometimes unjustified)	Blood loss	Surgical resections (reduced absorptive surface)
	Depression	Steatorrhea	
	Medication	Exudative enteropathy	

Perhaps one of the main causes of malnutrition in IBD patients is increased nutrient loss since intestinal transit of nutrients is considerably shortened. Multiple diarrhoic episodes sometimes immediately after eating accompanied by vomiting and/or occult/overt blood loss are responsible for the loss of the valuable micro- and macronutrients, fluids and electrolytes. Exudative enteropathy on the other hand can lead to excess protein loss.

Depression due to disease activity and severe restrictions in social life or working ability can play a significant role in the emergence of malnutrition because of appetite loss. (Table 1)

Nutritional Assessment and Anthropometry

A higher incidence of malnutrition has been historically reported in studies performed more than 30 years ago. Severely diseased patients have been treated for extended periods with corticosteroids unable to be weaned of them since the therapeutic options in those times were limited mainly to 5-Aminosalicylicate acids (5-ASA), corticosteroids and immunosupressants (Harries 1983, Fernandez-Banarez 1989). The past decade treatment options differ substantially since the introduction of the anti-Tumor Necrosis Factors in 1998 in the US and in 1999 in Europe for CD and in 2006 for UC. The combined therapy with anti-TNFs and immunosupressants Azathioprine/6 Mercaptopurine or Methotrexate or monotherapy with immunosupressants or immunomodulators have offered to IBD patients long periods of clinical and endoscopic relapse (Colombel 2010). Therefore the correlation between disease activity and nutritional deficiency differs from that of the past since although evident malnutrition may not be that often encountered nutritional deficiencies are almost always present and should be carefully examined.

Sousa Guerreiro et al have evaluated the nutritional status between 78 patients with inactive or mildly active Crohn's disease and 80 healthy controls. Mean Body Mass Index was lower in IBD patients but a striking 32% and 8% of CD patients versus 33,8% and 23,8% of controls were overweight (BMI>25) and obese (BMI>30) respectively. Several dietary restrictions among CD patients resulted in lower consumption of grains, milk, vegetables and fruits. As a result CD patients received lower daily intakes of Calcium, vitamins K, C, E, carbohydrates and monounsaturated fats (Sousa Guerreiro 2007). It seems therefore challenging to establish a validated method of nutritional assessment for these patients since standard BMI does not seem to provide enough clinical evidence regarding the level of nutritional deficiencies in micro- and micronutrients. Even overweight or obese patients present with specific nutrient deficiencies which are related to the exclusion of certain food types from their diet. This practice may be initially recommended by their treating physicians during disease flares and may be extended by patients in disease-free periods.

On the other hand, malnutrition in the form of obesity is not rare in the era of immunomodulators (Steed 2009). Since obesity is nowadays considered a chronic inflammatory state by the production of TNF-a and IL-6 it may aggravate or perpetuate the enhanced inflammatory response in CD and UC patients (Murch 1998, Cancello 2006, Fresno 2011, Procaccini 2011).

Mijac et al propose a simple and cost-effective method for routine nutritional assessment for IBD patients during their scheduled clinical visits. Measurement of BMI and serum albumin provide enough evidence regarding nutrient consumption and the nutritional status (Mijac 2010).

Table 2. Methods of evaluation of the nutritional status in IBD patients

BMI
Anthropometry
Serum Albumin
DEXA
Hand grip strength

DEXA: Dual Energy X-ray Absorptiometry (for bone density measurement).

Common anthropometric parameters could be used for the evaluation of malnutrition. Although BMI is reported as the first indication of malnutrition this may not be the case in these obese malnourished patients. Other anthropometric parameters should be also evaluated. Mid arm muscle circumference and mid arm circumference, triceps skinfold thickness, biceps skinfold thickness are common anthropometric measurements which can contribute to a better understanding of the nutritional status of IBD patients because they are commonly affected in the active phase of the disease but they are of limited use (Valentini 2011). Geerling et al have observed a decrease in power and endurance in the flexor muscles of CD patients reflecting the gradual loss of muscle strength. However, fat mass and free fat mass are also reported to be decreased especially in males (Geerling 2000). In this context Valentini et al report apart from a decrease in handgrip strength as a functional measurement of their nutritional state, a decreased body cell mass even in the 2/3 of UC and CD patients who are regarded well nourished (Valentini 2008). (Tables 2,3)

Table 3. Anthropometric measurements

Weight (kg)	BMI (kg/m^2) = weight (or estimated dry weight) / $(height)^2$
Height (cm)	MAMC (cm) = MAC – (TSF x π)
MAC (cm)	MAA (mm^2) = (π/4) x (MAC/π)
TST (mm)	MAMA (mm^2) = $(MAC-(\pi \times TST))^2 / 4\pi$
	MAFA (mm^2) = MAA - MAMA

BMI: Body mass index, MAMC: mid arm muscle circumference, MAC: mid arm circumference, TST: Triceps skinfold thickness, π: 3,142, MAA: Mid arm area, MAMA: mid arm muscle area, MAFA: Mid arm fat area.

When to Intervene and How

Nutritional intervention may play a significant role in the management of inflammatory bowel diseases as a whole. Multiple nutrient deficiencies are observed in IBD patients even in disease-free periods. It is not unusual to find anemia and hypoalbuminemia, deficiencies in minerals such as iron, zinc, copper, magnesium, calcium, phosphorus and vitamins such as vitamins A, B12, C, E, D, K. Megaloblastic anemia as a result of folic acid depletion and niacin deficiency may be present.

IBD patients represent a heterogeneous population with different needs regarding nutritional support. CD patients seem to be more prone to malnutrition since the absorptive epithelium is more severely affected than that of UC patients by inflammation, strictures, blind loops and fistulae. The nutritional status during disease flares differs substantially from that of patients in remission and can be aggravated during long lasting and therapy refractory disease periods.

It is therefore crucial to determine when and how to intervene in each patient individually in order to alter the disease sequence and maybe the outcome and to ameliorate the possible visible effects of nutritional deficiencies. Nutrition as induction of remission in CD patients with or without the use of other medication and on the other edge nutrition as maintenance therapy are two possible therapeutic interventions that may play a crucial role in disease control. The form of nutritional support may involve enteral nutrition exclusively or complementary, total parenteral nutrition or dietary guidance. (Table 4)

Table 4. Nutritional interventions: Means of nutritional intervention as therapeutic measurements for the induction and maintenance of clinical remission and correction of the nutritional deficits

Specific oral diet
Enteral nutrition
Parenteral nutrition
Correction of micronutrient deficits
Alternative therapies

A) Enteral Nutrition (EN) for Induction of Remission in Adults with Crohn's Disease

Enteral nutrition in the form of exclusive diet or supplementary, with a proportion of the daily energy intake provided orally, has been proved to have significant effect on the improvement of the nutritional status and the induction of mucosal healing in CD patients (Royall 1995, Fell 2000). These positive outcomes have significant impact on the disease outcome since deep mucosal healing is a predictor of prolonged clinical remission (Travis 2011). EN can induce clinical remission and in some trials reaches the effects of corticosteroids. In a Cochrane Database meta-analysis (Zachos 2008) the efficacy of EN versus corticosteroids was examined. 192 patients on EN and 160 patients on steroids were included in the meta-analysis. An OR of 0,33 favoring steroid therapy (95% CI: 0,21-0,53) was yielded but the relapse rates among patients in clinical remission at 12 months were similar, 65% in EN and 67% on steroids. Nevertheless it is improper to compare two therapeutic modalities with different mechanisms of action and safety profiles. The well known side effects of prolonged steroid therapy and the insignificant side effects of EN are matters of serious consideration and therefore although steroids are more effective in achieving clinical remission the need for prolonged and multiple periods of treatment make EN somehow more attractive as treatment modality.

According to the The second European evidence-based consensus on the diagnosis and management of Crohn's disease in 2010: "enteral therapy is regarded as only appropriate for adjunctive treatment to support nutrition and not for primary therapy. It is generally considered appropriate to induce remission only for patients who decline other drug therapy." (Dignass 2010)

The nitrogen source of enteral nutrition formulas can be classified as elemental (free amino acids), semi-elemental (oligopeptides) and polymeric (whole protein). There seems to be no difference in efficacy between elemental and polymeric diets. Formula compositions in general do not differ regarding their efficacy and since elemental diets are unpalatable and may lead to therapy drop outs, they should not be preferred over polymeric diets. (Akobeng 2000, Zachos 2007)

The fat content of EN diets, low fat <20g/1000kCal vs high fat >20g/1000kCal does not seem to alter the results of EN on clinical remission. Diets with very low fat content (0,6-1,3% of total calories) may be more efficient (Gorard 2003). Very low fat (<10%) long chain triglyceride diet content has also been demonstrated to favor clinical outcome vs low fat (>10%) long chain triglyceride diet content, but without significant statistical difference. Investigators based their studies on the hypothesis that fat content in diet could alter the production of anti-inflammatory cytokines, but larger trials are required to draw statistically significant results before treatment guidelines are issued. (Leiper 2001, Sakurai 2002, Gassull 2002, Bamba 2003)

Carbohydrate content is similar in most EN formulations and therefore no results can be drawn regarding the effect of carbohydrate content on remission in IBD.

Enrichment of EN formulations with bioactive peptides such as omega -3 fatty acids, glutamine, butyrate, antioxidants and TGF-β2 does not enhance the therapeutic outcome. (Geerling 2000, Macdonald 2006)

The mechanism of action of EN on CD remains unknown. Bannerjee et al have demonstrated that EN may exert its' mechanism of action through an anti-inflammatory effect (Bannerjee 2004). A reduction of IL-6 and a rise in IGF-1 in pediatric CD patients receiving a polymeric diet may be responsible for the clinical remission demonstrated in this group of patients.

Disease duration and location do not influence treatment outcomes in patients on EN. Although a trend towards favorable results when the small intestine is involved was shown by Afzal et al, more data are required for confirmation (Afzal 2004).

Side effects of enteral nutrition are rare and minimal in importance. Borreli et al report nausea, abdominal pain, flatulence and diarrhea as the side effects reported on exclusive enteral nutrition (Borrelli 2006).

B) Enteral Nutrition as Maintenance Therapy in Adults with Crohn's Disease

Achieving clinical and endoscopic remission with the use of EN formulations is certainly a very different treatment goal than maintaining clinical remission. Prevention of clinical relapse and avoidance of therapeutic options such as corticosteroids is sometimes challenging. In a study conducted by Takagi et al 51 CD patients in clinical remission were randomly assigned to receive half of their dietary calories in the form of an elemental EN formula or an unrestricted diet. The group of patients on EN presented a much lower relapse rate (34%) than the group with an unrestricted diet (64%) (OR 0,3, 95% CI: 0,09-0,94) (Takagi 2006). Endoscopic recurrence after surgical resection for ileal or ileocolonic CD was evaluated by Yamamoto et al in patients randomly assigned to receive supplementary enteral diet or unrestricted diet. Six months after the operation relapse rate among the EN patients was 25% whereas among the patients on unrestricted diet was 40% and 12 months after the operation 30% and 70% respectfully (Yamamoto 2007).

Both elemental and polymeric diets are equally effective in maintaining remission after induction therapy with corticosteroids or other therapeutic options and may provide a useful therapeutic tool in the effort to withdraw a patient from corticosteroid treatment.

C) Parenteral Nutrition (PN) in Adults with Crohn's Disease

During the eighties patients were assigned to receive parenteral nutrition as salvage therapy for avoidance of surgical excisions in severe and debilitating clinical relapses with good but temporary results. The patients relapsed shortly after the cessation of PN requiring further treatment. Nowadays PN can become useful for nutritional support in severely malnourished patients and as supportive therapy pre- and post- operatively. Serious complications while on PN are often and maybe life threatening. Infusion related sepsis and biliary complications are often encountered and may lead to hospitalizations. However the patients requiring parenteral nutrition, sometimes for long periods, experience an improvement of their nutritional status, their quality of life and may in some cases achieve clinical remission.

D) Enteral or Parenteral Nutrition for Induction of Remission and as Maintenance Therapy in Adults with Ulcerative Colitis

According to the guidelines of the ECCO consensus on UC "Enteral or parenteral nutritional therapy is inappropriate primary treatment …and … there is no indication for a special diet" However nutritional assessment should be performed whenever necessary and nutritional support should be provided (Stange 2008). Bowel rest and nutritional support may justify the use of total parenteral nutrition as adjunctive therapy in cases of toxic megacolon, ileus or subileus but is not often necessary.

E) Micronutrients Recommendations for IBD Patients

Nutritional deficiencies in micronutrients are evident in the majority of IBD patients even in clinical remission (Hébuterne 2009). They usually occur early in the disease process and are often underecognized due to the challenging therapeutic interventions that are required during disease onset and flares and the attention that is drawn in these efforts by treating physicians.

Table 5. Micronutrients recommendations for IBD patients

Iron 60 mg/d Supplemental elemental Fe, preferably ferrous sulphate or ferrous gluconate
Calcium 1000 mg/day Calcium carbonate with vitamin D
Vitamin D Cholecalciferol 800 IU/d or calcidiol 50 mg/d
Docosahexaenoic acid and eicosapentaenoic acid 1 g/d (to lower the use of anti-inflammatory Drugs)
Magnesium 300mg elemental Mg/d. Magnesium oxide provides 60% elemental Mg, magnesium chloride and lactate, with a lower Mg content (12%) has higher bioavailability
Folic acid 800 mg/d
Vitamin B-12 Patients with severe ileal disease 1 mg/d orally or parenteral vitamin B-12

(Moorthy et al 2008).

The therapeutic priorities may not entail nutritional correction of micronutrient deficiencies but it is noteworthy that proper correction of these deficiencies may benefit the general clinical outcome, may prevent severe complications such as anemia, osteopenia and osteoporosis which may have an adverse effect on the general well being of the patients and their chance of prolonged clinical remission. Moorthy et al have proposed specific recommendations regarding the correction of micronutrient deficiencies and prevention of anemia and bone loss in IBD patients (Moorthy 2008). Since many of these patients receive corticosteroids it is prudent to suggest proper supplementation of micronutrients because osteopenia and osteoporosis are well known side effects of therapy on corticosteroids. (Table 5)

Malnutrition in Children with IBD

The pediatric population of inflammatory bowel diseases represents a group of patients with different disease pattern and special needs regarding nutrition and growth. It is of great importance to mention that up to 90% of children present weight loss at diagnosis (Seidman 1991). Griffins et al report a 50-65% weight loss in children with UC and in 85% in children with CD (Griffiths 1993). In an study of 783 newly diagnosed children 22-24% with CD and 7-9% with UC presented with very low BMI of $<5^{th}$ percentile and an interesting 10% and 20-30% of CD and UC patients were reported to be overweight reflecting the new trend towards obesity as the new form of malnutrition in our times similar to that for the adults (Kugathasan 2007).

Since CD and UC are chronic diseases with periods of clinical relapse and remission, lasting for the entire lifetime of patients current therapies should focus not only to the alleviation of symptoms and to mucosal healing but to the correction of nutritional deficiencies which can have a major effect on growth. Growth failure and retardation are commonly seen among children and adolescents with CD, situation which may be the first clinical sign of the disease even before the onset of gastrointestinal symptoms (Sentongo 2000). The aetiopathogenesis of growth failure is multifactorial and poorly understood. IL-6 seems to play a significant role in growth impairment representing 40% of all probable causes of this disease complication. Another theory supports the disturbance of the growth hormone/insulin like growth factor axis. The mean final height of 123 CD patients with disease diagnosis at childhood and early puberty was 2,4 cm less than the parental or target height (range -20 to +9cm). In this study it is interesting to mention that the use of corticosteroids and surgical excisions were not linked to the impaired linear growth. The most important factor recognized as responsible for growth retardation were disease in the jejunum and the period of symptoms prior to disease diagnosis (Sawczenko 2006).

Nutritional intervention plays a dual role in pediatric IBD: prevention of growth retardation and a primary therapeutic role either for induction of remission or maintenance therapy. EN vs corticosteroids trials have yielded interesting results regarding growth in children with IBD. Height was significantly increased in the EN arms of the trials (Thomas 1993). A study of pediatric CD treated with the immunomodulator infliximab demonstrated an improvement of height velocity and height percentiles when the medication was introduced early in the course of the disease and before puberty. The use of 6-Mercaptopurine or growth hormone had no effect on linear growth and cannot be recommended (Heuschkel 2008).

Exclusive enteral nutrition (EEN) as induction therapy has been extensively studied in the pediatric population. EEN represents the use of elemental or polymeric enteral feeding formulas which replace normal diet as a distinct form of therapy, orally or through a self inserted nasogastric tube, until remission is achieved. A meta-analysis of five studies involving 147 children with CD which were assigned to exclusive EN concluded that EEN had equal effects on induction of remission with corticosteroids but with fewer side effects (Heuschkel 2000). These studies demonstrate a great difference between the pediatric and adult population in respect of EEN vs corticosteroids as primary therapies for induction of remission. Pediatric Crohn's Disease Activity Index (PCDAI) scores and C-reactive protein (CRP) decreased promptly after EEN and in some cases mood and energy improved (Day 2006, Bannerjee 2004). Borrelli et al report that mucosal healing was present in 74% of children receiving EEN for 10 weeks while only 33% of the steroid treated patients exhibited endoscopic remission and mucosal healing. PCDAI score, erythrocyte sedimentation rates, CRP decreased and serum albumin levels increased. Therefore the pediatric population of IBD patients are ideal candidates for EN as induction and maintenance therapy as the disease sequence is certainly altered and growth retardation may be prevented (Borrelli 2006).

Conclusion

The primary goals in inflammatory bowel diseases are induction of remission, avoidance of disease flares and maintenance of clinical and endoscopic remission. Nevertheless nutritional evaluation and correction of nutritional deficiencies should become one of the major therapeutic interventions in IBD patients since it can further contribute to mucosal healing, clinical remission and may improve health related quality of life. General and non specific dietary restrictions may not contribute to avoidance of disease flares but on the contrary may aggravate the nutritional status of IBD patients with multiple clinical implications. However the pathophysiology of malnutrition in IBD is multifactorial and not completely clarified. The majority of patients present at onset, during severe disease flares, some form of malnutrition. The severely malnourished patient with CD with severely affected BMI, depletion of body cell mass and electrolyte abnormalities may not be encountered that often in the era of immunomodulators and proper medical management but is still there and can become a challenge regarding the nutritional support required. Enteral nutrition is the modality of choice in severe cases but it has been proposed as induction therapy with or without medications and as maintenance therapy supplementary with oral diet. The different concentrations in fat, protein, carbohydrates and bioactive peptides are of no clinical importance regarding the clinical outcome since they all produce the same results. A small favorable trend towards very low in fat diets may exist. Children and adolescents with IBD may benefit more than adults from EN, exclusive or supplementary. EN can be an alternative therapeutic modality to medication therapy for pediatric IBD, as induction or maintenance therapy. Growth retardation could be prevented with proper nutritional guidance. Parenteral nutrition on the other hand is restricted to the few cases where bowel rest is required in both diseases and is not recommended for induction of remission or as maintenance therapy. An increased clinical awareness regarding early recognition of malnutrition in IBD in conjunction with proper therapeutic nutritional intervention may improve the nutritional status of IBD patients, fact that could have a positive effect on disease outcome, mucosal healing and quality of life.

REFERENCES

Afzal NA, Van Der Zaag-Loonen HJ, Arnaud-Battandier F, Davies S, Murch S, Derkx B, Heuschkel R, Fell JM. Improvement in quality of life *Aliment Pharmacol. Ther*. 2004 15;20(2):167-172.

Akobeng AK, Miller V, Stanton J, Elbadri AM, Thomas AG. Double-blind randomized controlled trial *J. Pediatr. Gastroenterol. Nutr.* 2000;30(1):78-84.

Ballinger A, El-Haj T, Perrett D, Turvill J, Obeid O, Dryden S, Williams G, Farthing MJ. The role of medial hypothalamic serotonin in the suppression of feeding in a rat model of colitis. *Gastroenterology* 2000;118: 544-553.

Bamba T, Shimoyama T, Sasaki M, Tsujikawa T, Fukuda Y, Koganei K, Hibi T, Iwao Y, Munakata A, Fukuda S, Matsumoto T, Oshitani N, Hiwatashi N, Oriuchi T, Kitahora T, Utsunomiya T, Saitoh Y, Suzuki Y, Nakajima M. Dietary fat *Eur. J. Gastroenterol. Hepatol.* 2003;15(2):151-157.

Bannerjee K, Camacho-Hübner C, Babinska K, Dryhurst KM, Edwards R, Savage MO, Sanderson IR, Croft NM. Anti-inflammatory and growth *J. Pediatr. Gastroenterol. Nutr.* 2004;38(3):270-275.

Borrelli O, Cordischi L, Cirulli M, Paganelli M, Labalestra V, Uccini S, Russo PM, Cucchiara S. Polymeric diet *Clin. Gastroenterol. Hepatol.* 2006;4(6):744-753.

Cancello R, Clément K. Is obesity an inflammatory illness? Role of low-grade inflammation and macrophage infiltration in human white adipose tissue. *BJOG*. 2006;113(10):1141-1147.

Colombel JF, Sandborn WJ, Reinisch W, Mantzaris GJ, Kornbluth A, Rachmilewitz D, Lichtiger S, D'Haens G, Diamond RH, Broussard DL, Tang KL, van der Woude CJ, Rutgeerts P; SONIC Study Group. Infliximab, azathioprine, or combination therapy *N. Engl. J. Med.* 2010;362(15):1383-1395.

Day AS, Whitten KE, Lemberg DA, Clarkson C, Vitug-Sales M, Jackson R, Bohane TD. Exclusive enteral feeding as primary therapy *J. Gastroenterol. Hepatol.* 2006;21(10):1609-1614.

Dignass A, Van Assche G, Lindsay JO, Lémann M, Söderholm J, Colombel JF, Danese S, D'Hoore A, Gassull M, Gomollón F, Hommes DW, Michetti P, O'Morain C, Oresland T, Windsor A, Stange EF, Travis SP; European Crohn's and Colitis Organisation (ECCO). The second European evidence *J. Crohns. Colitis*. 2010;4(1):28-62.

Fell JM, Paintin M, Arnaud-Battandier F, Beattie RM, Hollis A, Kitching P, Donnet-Hughes A, MacDonald TT, Walker-Smith JA. Mucosal healing and a fall in mucosal pro-inflammatory cytokine mRNA induced by a specific oral polymeric diet in paediatric Crohn's disease. *Aliment Pharmacol. Ther.* 2000;14: 281-289.

Fernandez-Banares F, Abad-Lacruz A, Xiol X, Gine JJ, Dolz C, Cabre E, Esteve M, Gonzalez-Huix F, Gassull MA. Vitamin status in patients with inflammatory bowel disease. *Am. J. Gastroenterol.* 1989;84(7):744-748.

Fresno M, Alvarez R, Cuesta N. Toll-like receptors *Arch. Physiol. Biochem.* 2011; doi:10.3109/13813455. 2011.562514.

Gassull MA, Fernández-Bañares F, Cabré E, Papo M, Giaffer MH, Sánchez-Lombraña JL, Richart C, Malchow H, González-Huix F, Esteve M; Eurpoean Group on Enteral Nutrition in Crohn's Disease. Fat composition may be a clue to explain the primary therapeutic effect of enteral nutrition in Crohn's disease: results of a double blind randomised multicentre *European trial. Gut.* 2002;51(2):164-168.

Geerling BJ, Badart-Smook A, Stockbrügger RW, Brummer RJ. Comprehensive nutritional status *Eur. J. Clin. Nutr.* 2000;54(6):514-521.

Geerling BJ, Badart-Smook A, van Deursen C, van Houwelingen AC, Russel MG, Stockbrugger RW, Brummer RJ. Nutritional supplementation with N-3 fatty acids and antioxidants in patients with Crohn's disease in remission: effects on antioxidant status and fatty acid profile. *Inflamm. Bowel Dis.* 2000;6:77-84.

Gorard DA. Enteral nutrition in Crohn's disease: fat in the formula. *Eur. J. Gastroenterol. Hepatol.* 2003;15:115-118.

Griffiths AM, Nguyen P, Smith C, MacMillan JH, Sherman PM.

Growth and clinical course of children *Gut.* 1993;34(7):939-943.

Harries AD, Heatley RV. Nutritional disturbances in Crohn's disease. *Postgrad Med. J.* 1983;59(697):690-697.

Hartman C, Eliakim R, Shamir R. Nutritional status and nutritional therapy *World J. Gastroenterol.* 2009;15(21):2570-2578.

Hébuterne X, Filippi J, Al-Jaouni R, Schneider S. Nutritional consequences and nutrition *Gastroenterol. Clin. Biol.* 2009;33 Suppl 3:S235-244.

Heuschkel RB, Menache CC, Megerian JT, Baird AE. Enteral nutrition *J. Pediatr. Gastroenterol. Nutr.* 2000;31(1):8-15.

Heuschkel R, Salvestrini C, Beattie RM, Hildebrand H, Walters, Griffiths A. Guidelines for the management of growth failure in childhood inflammatory bowel disease. *Inflamm. Bowel Dis.* 2008;14(6):839-849.

Jowett SL, Seal CJ, Phillips E, Gregory W, Barton JR, Welfare MR. Dietary beliefs of people with ulcerative colitis *Clin. Nutr.* 2004;23(2):161-170.

Kugathasan S, Nebel J, Skelton JA, Markowitz J, Keljo D, Rosh J, LeLeiko N, Mack D, Griffiths A, Bousvaros A, Evans J, Mezoff A, Moyer S, Oliva-Hemker M, Otley A, Pfefferkorn M, Crandall W, Wyllie R, Hyams J. Body mass index in children with newly diagnosed inflammatory bowel disease: observations from two multicenter North American inception cohorts. *J. Pediatr.* 2007;151: 523-527.

Kupcinskas L, Lakatos PL, Mantzaris GJ, Schreiber S, Villanacci V, Warren BF; for the European Crohn's and Colitis Organisation (ECCO). European evidence-based Consensus on the diagnosis and management of ulcerative colitis: Definitions and diagnosis. *J. Crohns. Colitis*. 2008;2(1):1-23.

Lanfranchi GA, Brignola C, Campieri M, Bazzocchi G, Pasquali R, Bassein L, Labo G. Assessment of nutritional status in Crohn's disease in remission or low activity. *Hepatogastroenterology* 1984; 31:129-132.

Leiper K, Woolner J, Mullan MM, Parker T, van der Vliet M, Fear S, Rhodes JM, Hunter JO. A randomised controlled trial *Gut*. 2001;49(6):790-794.

Macdonald A. Omega-3 fatty acids *Gastroenterol. Nurs*. 2006;29(4):295-301.

Mijac DD, Janković GL, Jorga J, Krstić MN Nutritional status in patients with active inflammatory bowel *Eur. J. Intern. Med.* 2010;21(4):315-319.

Moorthy D, Cappellano KL, Rosenberg IH. Nutrition and Crohn's disease: an update of print and Web-based guidance. Nutr Rev. 2008;66(7):387-397.

Murch SH. Local and systemic effects of macrophage cytokines in intestinal inflammation. *Nutrition* 1998;14:780-783.

Procaccini C, Carbone F, Galgani M, La Rocca C, De Rosa V, Cassano S, Matarese G. Obesity and susceptibility *Expert Rev. Clin. Immunol.* 2011;7(3):287-294.

Royall D, Greenberg GR, Allard JP, Baker JP, Jeejeebhoy KN. Total enteral nutrition support improves body composition of patients with active Crohn's disease. *JPEN J. Parenter. Enteral Nutr*. 1995;19: 95-99.

Sakurai T, Matsui T, Yao T, Takagi Y, Hirai F, Aoyagi K, Okada M. Short-term efficacy of enteral nutrition *JPEN J. Parenter. Enteral. Nutr*. 2002;26(2):98-103.

Sawczenko A, Ballinger AB, Savage MO, Sanderson IR. Clinical features affecting final adult height in patients with pediatric-onset Crohn's disease. *Pediatrics* 2006;118(1):124-129.

Seidman E, LeLeiko N, Ament M, Berman W, Caplan D, Evans J, Kocoshis S, Lake A, Motil K, Sutphen J. Nutritional issues in pediatric inflammatory bowel disease. *J. Pediatr. Gastroenterol. Nutr*. 1991;12: 424-438.

Sentongo TA, Semeao EJ, Piccoli DA, Stallings VA, Zemel BS. Growth, body composition, and nutritional status in children and adolescents with Crohn's disease. *J. Pediatr. Gastroenterol. Nutr.* 2000;31:33-40.

Sousa Guerreiro C, Cravo M, Costa AR, Miranda A, Tavares L, Moura-Santos P, MarquesVidal P, Nobre Leitao C. A comprehensive approach to evaluate nutritional status in Crohn's patients in the era of biologic therapy: a casecontrol study. *Am. J. Gastroenterol*. 2007; 102:2551-2556.

Stange EF, Travis SP, Vermeire S, Reinisch W, Geboes K, Barakauskiene A, Feakins R, Fléjou JF, Herfarth H, Hommes DW, Kupcinskas L, Lakatos PL, Mantzaris GJ, Schreiber S, Villanacci V, Warren BF; for the

European Crohn's and Colitis Organisation (ECCO). European evidence-based Consensus on the diagnosis and management of ulcerative colitis: Definitions and diagnosis. *J. Crohns Colitis* 2008;2(1):1-23.

Steed H, Walsh S, Reynolds N. A brief report of the epidemiology *Obes. Facts* 2009;2(6):370-372.

Takagi S, Utsunomiya K, Kuriyama S, Yokoyama H, Takahashi S, Iwabuchi M, Takahashi H, Takahashi S, Kinouchi Y, Hiwatashi N, Funayama Y, Sasaki I, Tsuji I, Shimosegawa T. Effectiveness of an 'half elemental diet' as maintenance therapy for Crohn's disease: A randomized-controlled trial. *Aliment Pharmacol. Ther*. 2006;24: 1333-1340.

Tanaka M, Shibayama T, Sato E, Sasaki S, Kazuma K. Dietary intake and body composition of Japanese ulcerative colitis patients in remission. *Gastroenterol. Nurs.* 2007;30(5):357-362.

Thomas AG, Taylor F, Miller V. Dietary intake and nutritional treatment in childhood Crohn's disease. *J. Pediatr. Gastroenterol. Nutr.* 1993;17: 75-81.

Travis SP, Higgins PD, Orchard T, Van Der Woude CJ, Panaccione R, Bitton A, O'Morain C, Panés J, Sturm A, Reinisch W, Kamm MA, D'Haens G. Review article: defining remission in ulcerative colitis. *Aliment Pharmacol. Ther.* 2011;doi:10.1111/j.1365-2036.2011.04701.x.

Valentini L, Schaper L, Buning C, Hengstermann S, Koernicke T, Tillinger W, Guglielmi FW, Norman K, Buhner S, Ockenga J, Pirlich M, Lochs H. Malnutrition and impaired muscle strength *Nutrition* 2008;24(7-8):694-702.

Valentini L, Schulzke JD. Mundane, yet challenging: the assessment of malnutrition in inflammatory bowel disease. *Eur. J. Intern. Med.* 2011;22(1):13-15.

Van Patter WN, Bargen JA, Dockerty MB, Feldman WH, Mayo CW, Waugh JM. Regional enteritis. *Gastroenterology* 1954;26:347-450.

Yamamoto T, Nakahigashi M, Umegae S, Kitagawa T, Matsumoto K. Impact of long-term enteral nutrition *Aliment Pharmacol. Ther*. 2007;25(1):67-72.

Zachos M, Tondeur M, Griffiths AM. Enteral nutritional therapy for induction of remission in Crohn's disease. *Cochrane Database Syst. Rev.* 2007;(1):CD000542.

Zoli G, Katelaris PH, Garrow J, Gasbarrini G, Farthing MJ. Increased energy expenditure in growing adolescents with Crohn's disease. *Dig. Dis. Sci.* 1996;41:1754-1759.

In: Malnutrition: Risk Factors …
Editor: J.B. Knudsen
ISBN: 978-1-62100-351-9

Chapter 4

THE TOLERANCE MODEL: A NON-INFLAMMATORY FORM OF IMMUNE COMPETENCE PREVAILS IN ACUTE PRE-PUBESCENT MALNUTRITION

Bill Woodward and Jennifer M. Monk
Department of Human Health and Nutritional Sciences,
University of Guelph, Ontario, Canada

ABSTRACT

Depressed inflammatory immune competence is characteristic of acute (i.e., wasting) protein and energy deficits in pre-pubescent humans and animals, and a substantial catalogue of clinical and experimental information has grown up around this classic observation. Unfortunately, however, the conceptual underpinning for the subject has not kept pace. Thus, the inflammatory decline associated with acute malnutrition continues to be seen in surprisingly simplistic terms as a component of a generalized and unregulated process of immunological disintegration pursuant to weight loss and limited substrate supply. This paradigm reflects a view of the malnutrition-associated immune system as an isolated silo without reference to other physiological systems or to the endocrine governance of metabolism. Although sufficient to launch the research front of nutritional immunology, such an unphysiological model cannot stimulate a scholarly development of the subject to productive maturity. Significantly, therefore, a new and more sophisticated concept has emerged, stemming from the point of view that any physiological change associated with acute malnutrition represents an attempt to adapt and, thus, is a regulated phenomenon conferring benefits in the face of a limited availability of energy and substrates.

Endocrinological and metabolic evidence is available of adaptive attempts extending even into the advanced stages of wasting disease in both clinical and experimental settings. In turn, this information base provides a framework within which to incorporate a body of immunological findings that defies the prevailing disintegrative paradigm but is easily accommodated by a newly-proposed adaptive, or regulative, model. The critical immunological evidence derives mainly from experimental animal studies of acute malnutrition in its more advanced stages and centers on studies of several cytokines that play key roles in defining the fundamental character of immune competence. As a consequence the proposition has emerged that acute pre-pubescent protein and energy deficit stimulates an immunological re-orientation emphasizing a non-inflammatory and tolerogenic form of immune competence. Such an adaptation may reduce the risk of autoimmune pathologies in response to a flood of catabolically-released self-antigens, but would do so at the expense of an increased susceptibility to opportunistic infection. This proposition, dubbed the Tolerance Model, provides a foundation both for renewed scholarly vigour in the study of malnutrition-associated immune competence and for optimism with respect to management prospects for the most debilitated clinical cases.

1. INTRODUCTION

Up to two million largely infection-related deaths occur annually among children under five years of age suffering from acute primary deficits of protein and energy, and this toll is undoubtedly exceeded by the additional burden of infection-related morbidity [1]. Both acute (i.e., wasting) and stunting forms of primary protein-energy malnutrition increase the risk of childhood mortality in a potent multiplicative manner as the severity of nutritional deficit increases [2]. The most widely-recognized relationship between pre-pubescent protein-energy malnutrition and infection is the synergism expressed in the classic concept of the Malnutrition-Infection Cycle [3], and the depiction shown in Figure 1 reflects the acceptance of immune depression as a determining factor in the infection-related morbidity and mortality of childhood malnutrition. Data pertaining to stunting malnutrition and immune defences are scant but suggestive, whereas information relating acute (i.e., wasting) malnutrition to immune competence is abundant, although skewed toward grade 3 disease [3]. In this chapter the term "malnutrition", when used without qualification, refers to acute forms of protein and energy deficit. It should be noted that between 40 and 70% of critically ill children exhibit secondary malnutrition and high susceptibility to infection [4], and there is every reason to expect that the relationship embodied in the Malnutrition-Infection Cycle applies also to this form of pathology.

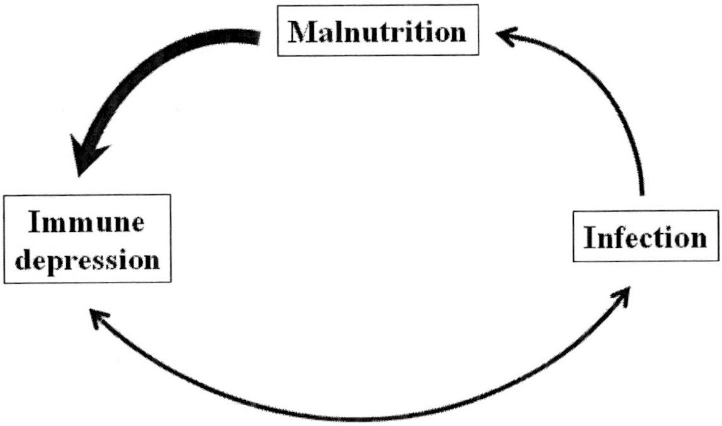

Figure 1. The Malnutrition-Infection Cycle depicted for acute deficits of protein and energy and showing immune depression as an essential component. The bolded arrow highlights the part of the cycle on which the most research effort has been concentrated. A bidirectional connection links infection and immune depression because many infections that are aggravated by malnutrition also reduce classic immune competence.

As reviewed elsewhere [3], a substantial catalogue of clinical and experimental observations has established that an attenuated inflammatory response, whether primarily innate or adaptive in nature, is characteristic of acute childhood malnutrition. In turn, this phenomenon is widely interpreted to reflect a chaotic process of immunological disintegration consequent to inadequate metabolic supplies of substrates, especially nitrogenous compounds, and energy [3]. A more sophisticated paradigm, however, is needed to accommodate the full range of evidence relating malnutrition and inflammatory immune competence, and a concept dubbed the Tolerance Model [5-9] has emerged to fulfill this role. According to this proposition, malnutrition elicits a tightly regulated immunological reconfiguration in an effort to sustain a predominantly non-inflammatory form of immune competence. Because acute malnutrition releases a flood of potentially inflammatory self-antigens [10, 11], the presumptive primary benefit is a reduced risk of damaging autoimmune reactions. Interestingly, this adaptive component of the model was proposed initially more than twenty years ago [12] and, subsequently, was put forward independently twelve years later [13]. At the same time the model acknowledges, and predicts (as a consequence of reduced inflammatory competence), the susceptibility to opportunistic infection that is a consistent feature of acute, pre-pubescent malnutrition. This chapter identifies the main planks in the platform of the Tolerance Model.

2. A Non-Inflammatory Mediator Profile Prevails in Acute Malnutrition

Depressed inflammatory competence is the most consistent immunological feature of acute pediatric malnutrition, and is the basis for the essentially universal conclusion that acute malnutrition causes immune depression [3]. Oddly, although non-inflammatory immune competence is well-known [14], this component of systemic immune defence has not been incorporated formally into the conceptual framework relating malnutrition and immunology.

The glucocorticoid hormones together with transforming growth factor(TGF)-β and interleukin(IL)-10 comprise a partially redundant anti-inflammatory triad widely regarded as the backbone of peripheral self-tolerance [15-17]. High blood levels of cortisol are a consistent feature of acute pediatric malnutrition in its advanced stages [18] and, extending this long-established observation, weanling rodent models of marasmus and incipient kwashiorkor exhibit blood serum levels of corticosterone which could be characterized as pharmacological [19]. In addition, extremely high blood bioactivities of TGF-β [5, 7, 20] and IL-10 [5, 6, 9] are reported in the advanced stages of weight loss in diverse animal models of acute, pre-pubescent malnutrition. Moreover, similar elevations in the blood concentrations of corticosterone, TGF-β and IL-10 are early features of weanling mouse pathologies that progress to mimic marasmus and kwashiorkor with fidelity [6, 7, 19]. Thus, blood concentrations of a potently anti-inflammatory triad of mediators rise early and are sustained in unison throughout the progression of wasting, pre-pubescent malnutrition. By contrast, low blood bioactivities of the potently inflammatory cytokine, interferon-γ, emerge simultaneously in the same weanling mouse models of marasmus and incipient kwashiorkor [21].

Blood concentrations of endocrine hormones and cytokines represent spillover from the extravascular compartment and may be regarded as reflective of concentrations at extravascular sites of action [5, 22]. Moreover, blood levels of these mediators are particularly informative when assessed in panels to reflect "balance at the systemic level" [23]. Thus, a systemic non-inflammatory, or tolerogenic, mediator profile prevails in acute forms of pre-pubescent malnutrition. This does not suggest immune incompetence. Rather, it points to a new immunological set point emphasizing active, physiological support of a non-inflammatory form of competence.

3. Physiological Regulation is Sustained into Advanced Stages of Acute Malnutrition

3.1. Synthesis of Nitrogen-Containing Compounds

The thesis is developed elsewhere [3, 12] that malnutrition-associated immune depression is part of a larger attempt to adapt metabolically to acute deficits of protein and energy. As a point of logic, it follows that a coordinated metabolism specific to acute malnutrition must reflect continued metabolic control over physiological systems, including immune defences, while weight loss progresses. In this context, reports from two independent research groups, one pursuing a rodent model of acute malnutrition [24, 25] and the other studying human subjects [26], illustrate maintenance of metabolic control in the face of acute deficits of nitrogen and energy.

Straus et al. [24, 25] demonstrated fine control of hepatic protein synthesis in the acutely protein deficient weanling rat. In this experimental system, mRNA transcript levels of some proteins (albumin, transthyretin, carbamyl phosphate synthetase-I, class I alcohol dehydrogenase and insulin-like growth factor-1) decreased relative to total cellular RNA, whereas transcript levels of other proteins were either unaffected (ubiquitin and hypoxanthine-guanine phosphoribosyl transferase) or increased (H-ferritin and insulin-like growth factor binding proteins-1, -2 and -4). Further analysis produced evidence of regulation at the level of gene transcription.

Mayatepek et al. [26] reported a substantially similar phenomenon in relation to the synthesis of leukotrienes by acutely malnourished children. Leukotriene(LT)A_4 sits at a metabolic branchpoint such that it can give rise either to the inflammatory metabolite, LTB_4, or (through conjugation with glutathione) to the cysteine-containing metabolites, LTC_4, LTD_4 and LTE_4 [27]. It is not surprising, therefore, that glutathione deficiency secondary to congenital absence of glutathione synthetase results in a reduced capacity to synthesize cysteinyl leukotrienes [28]. In contrast, however, Mayatepek et al. [26] found depressed LTB_4 synthesis and increased synthesis of cysteinyl leukotrienes in vitro in the whole blood of children with kwashiorkor despite profound depression of erythrocyte glutathione levels in these subjects. Likewise, urinary LTE_4 excretion, an index of systemic synthesis of cysteinyl leukotrienes in vivo, was paradoxically high in the subjects with kwashiorkor relative to age- and sex-matched controls. In the same study, marasmic children gave evidence of a sustained capacity to synthesize cysteine-containing leukotrienes in vitro and in vivo despite apparent deficiency of glutathione as indicated by erythrocyte concentrations of this tripeptide.

Neither the studies of Straus et al. [24, 25] nor the report of Mayatepek et al. [26] can be accommodated within a model centered simplistically on a non-selective decrease in the synthesis of proteins and other amino acid-containing compounds in acute malnutrition. Rather, both groups appear to show that regulated apportionment of nitrogen according to wasting-associated metabolic priorities is sustained even in the most extreme forms of acute, pre-pubescent protein and energy deficits. It is reasonable to extrapolate this proposition to include nitrogen-based compounds critical to immune competence.

3.2. Systemic Endocrine Control and Metabolic Adaptation

The physiologic response to acute pre-pubescent malnutrition is orchestrated by endocrine hormones [18], and Figure 2 illustrates some major endocrine responses to acute pediatric protein and energy deficits as reflected by changes in blood hormonal concentrations that are characteristic of the advanced stages of weight loss. From a metabolic standpoint, this is an adaptive attempt aimed at conserving substrates and energy while promoting glucose homeostasis and the preferential use of fat as an energy source [18]. Because endocrine hormones govern the systemic distribution of substrates and energy in support of all physiological functions, it follows as a point of logic that wasting-associated immunobiology can be understood only within the context of the hormonally-mediated characteristics of wasting-associated metabolism. High glucocorticoid concentrations and low levels of both triiodothyronine (T_3) and leptin are implicated particularly clearly in the inflammatory immune depression that characterizes acute pre-pubescent malnutrition [3]. This evidence, centered on intervention studies using experimental animals, is summarized in the next section together with complementary information pertaining to cytokine-based interventions.

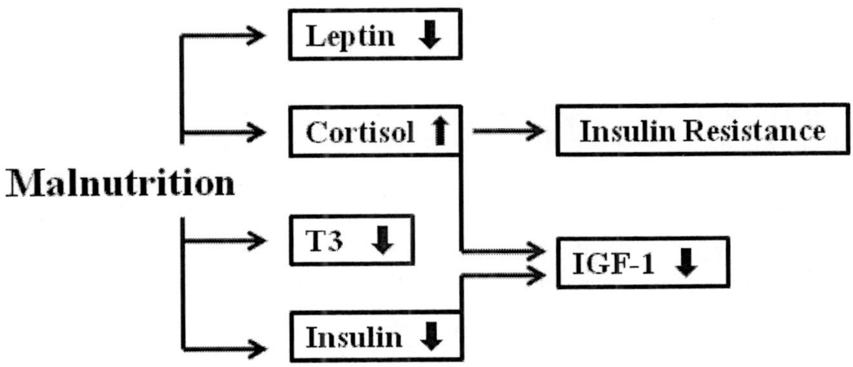

Figure 2. An outline of some adaptive endocrine responses to acute deficits of protein and energy, including some of the inter-relationships among these responses. Based on discussions by Pugliese [18], Ingenbleek [29] and Soliman et al. [30]. IGF-1, insulin-like growth factor-1; T3, triiodothyronine.

3.3. Responsiveness of Inflammatory Competence to Endocrine and Cytokine Interventions

Physiological systems are regulated by networks of hormonal and hormone-like mediators. Because of the interactive nature of their components, such networks present diverse points through which perturbation or intervention should yield a common physiological outcome. If regulation of inflammatory competence remains intact in acute malnutrition, therefore, one would predict responsiveness of inflammatory capacity to a diversity of soluble mediators.

The glucocorticoid hormones are potently anti-inflammatory [31], and one research group [32] has provided a glimpse of the immunological significance of high levels of these hormones in the acutely protein-deficient young adult mouse. In this investigation protein deficiency depressed the capacity of stimulated macrophages to perform inflammatory functions in vitro, whereas both adrenalectomy and administration of a glucocorticoid receptor antagonist abrogated this impact of dietary insufficiency. Importantly, the interventions did not influence food intake, weight change or plasma albumin concentrations and, hence, were effective in the face of unabated wasting malnutrition. Interestingly, intervention with injections of the cytokine, granulocyte-macrophage colony stimulating factor, achieved the same immunological outcome in this experimental system, also without influencing growth parameters or related biochemical indices [33].

T_3 is a component of the neuro-endocrine-immune axis [34, 35] and, despite a seemingly inconsistent literature, adaptive immune competence generally appears sub-optimal both in vivo and in vitro when T_3 concentrations are outside the physiological range. Nuclear T_3 receptors are reported in monocytes, peripheral lymphocytes, thymocytes, thymic epithelial cells and, most recently, in dendritic cells that exhibit the unique capacity for stimulating naïve T cells to elicit primary responses [35-37]. Although receptor numbers may be low in cells of the immunological periphery relative to receptor numbers in classical target cells [36], responsiveness to T_3 can be demonstrated in vitro [38]. Thus, the immunological influences of T_3 should be anticipated and may be exerted both directly and indirectly. More persuasively, depression in inflammatory humoral and cell-mediated immune competence was prevented [39-41], and depressed inflammatory humoral competence was reversed [42], by administration of exogenous T_3 to weanling mice subjected to acute malnutrition. Importantly, T_3 can exert these immunomodulatory influences in the acutely protein and energy deficient mouse independently of an impact on metabolic rate (according to the criteria of weight change, food intake and mobilization of fat and lean tissue) and despite exacerbated lymphoid involution [41].

Leptin is also implicated as a mediator of immune depression in acute deficits of protein and energy [43, 44]. The most intriguing evidence in this regard derives from studies of young adult mice sensitized during a 48-hour period of starvation to generate an inflammatory cell-mediated immune response [43]. In this model, exogenous leptin prevented development of depressed cell-mediated inflammatory competence without affecting either weight loss during the period of food deprivation and immune sensitization or subsequent catch-up growth during the period preceding immune challenge. A mechanistic basis for this finding derives from evidence identifying the naïve $CD4^+$ T cell as a target for leptin and showing that this hormone promotes a T cell cytokine production pattern, in vitro, that would be expected to favour inflammatory cell-mediated responses [43].

Fms-like tyrosine kinase 3 ligand (Flt3L) is a non-redundant cytokine that stimulates proliferation and differentiation of dendritic cells and their precursors and is both essential and sufficient for the homeostatic maintenance of dendritic cell compartments [45]. In turn, exogenous Flt3L expands dendritic cell populations of healthy murine and human recipients as does its conditional expression in experimental rodents [45]. Importantly, similar responsiveness in terms of cellular numbers was apparent in studies of the splenic dendritic cell compartment of acutely malnourished weanling mice given daily injections of recombinant murine Flt3L as wasting disease progressed [46]. Moreover, administration of the recombinant cytokine sustained inflammatory cell-mediated immune competence in the same experimental system in the face of unabated weight loss [46]. A basis for understanding the latter finding is provided by a report that dendritic cell numbers limit naïve T cell responses in vivo in the healthy adult mouse [47].

As illustrated by the foregoing summary, intervention studies spanning three endocrine hormones and two cytokines, three independent research groups and four distinct rodent models of malnutrition demonstrate prevention, or even reversal, of inflammatory immune depression in the face of ongoing weight loss [32, 33, 39-43, 46]. No dose-response information is available in this respect, but the key point is inescapable that responsiveness to multiple mediators is retained into the advanced stages of diverse forms of malnutrition. The studies relating to the glucocorticoids [32] provide functional information complementary to the compelling, but descriptive, reports of high blood glucocorticoid levels [18] in acute malnutrition, and similar intervention studies are required with respect to other inflammatory and non-inflammatory mediators for which blood concentration data are available, at present TGF-β [5, 7, 20], IL-10 [5, 6, 9] and interferon-γ [21]. In any case, this small body of evidence appears incompatible with a model of chaotic immunological disintegration, and requires a paradigm in which malnutrition elicits a tightly regulated, presumably purposeful, decline in inflammatory immune competence.

3.4. Expression of Cytokine Genes

Information pertaining to the expression of cytokine mRNA transcripts is available to complement the findings regarding the blood profile of bioactive mediator proteins. Thus, expression of IL-10 mRNA was elevated in mononuclear cells from the blood of children exhibiting various forms and degrees of acute malnutrition, whereas expression of mRNA for interferon-γ was simultaneously low [48]. Moreover, in mouse models of acute pediatric malnutrition, expression of mRNA for IL-10 and TGF-β1 increased several-fold in the spleen, a characteristically inflammatory site, while mRNA expression for the inflammatory cytokine, IL-12, specifically its p40 subunit, markedly declined [8]. Conversely, malnutrition exerted no influence on these indices in the small intestine, thus supporting the non-inflammatory character of this immunological organ. In both humans and animals, therefore, a picture emerges of cytokine gene expression reconfigured to sustain a non-inflammatory form of immune competence.

3.5. Systemic IL-10 Production in Vivo

A technique termed the in vivo cytokine capture assay permits assessment of the rate of cytokine production on a systemic level in an intact animal [49]. Briefly, the method centers on a biotin-conjugated monoclonal anti-cytokine antibody that is used to trap a small fraction of cytokine within the blood compartment. The accumulation of the resulting immune complex during a period of a few hours is subsequently quantified and, because blood cytokines represent spillover from their extravascular sources [21, 22], the capture assay provides an index that relates to production rate independently of cellular source [49, 50]. As discussed elsewhere [6, 9, 50], no in vivo index of cytokine production can be independent of physiological turnover. However, the capture assay traps newly-synthesized cytokine in an antibody complex that extends the typically brief half-life of the bound cytokine sufficiently to yield an index affected primarily by cytokine production rate. In effect, the method is a competitive binding procedure and an extension of the physiological phenomenon whereby the clearance of cytokines from the blood is retarded when these molecules form complexes with soluble cytokine receptors [51] or anti-cytokine autoantibodies [52].

The capture assay has been rigorously validated in the mouse for several cytokines including IFN-γ and IL-2, -4, -6 and -10 [49], and the assay has been applied to the expression of IL-10 by weanling mice subjected to acute malnutrition according to two distinct models, one a model of marasmus and the other mimicking incipient kwashiorkor. Constitutive production of IL-10 is at least sustained into the advanced stages of weight loss in both experimental systems [6, 9], and can exhibit elevation [6]. In apparent contrast, the capacity for challenge-induced production of IL-10 proved less robust than constitutive production of this cytokine in the face of acute malnutrition [9]. This finding is intriguing in view of the central tenet of the Tolerance Model that the primary physiological purpose of immune competence in acute malnutrition is to provide protection against self antigens rather than against external challenges. Moreover, the capacity to sustain challenge-induced production of IL-10 depends on the metabolic form of acute malnutrition and is independent of nitrogen or energy decrement [9], an outcome wholly incompatible with a paradigm of chaotic immunological disintegration but easily accommodated by a model centered on regulated immunological adaptation. It will be important to extend this evidence base to include assessments of systemic production of other key inflammation-related mediators.

3.6. Regulatory T Cells

The transcription factor, Foxp3, serves as a marker for major subsets of regulatory (i.e., anti-inflammatory) T cells of both thymic and peripheral origin [53]. It is of interest, therefore, that starvation sufficient to reduce cell-mediated inflammatory competence in the adult mouse nevertheless increased the proportion of $CD4^+$ T cells expressing Foxp3 [54]. Moreover, in complementary work, the expression of Foxp3 mRNA was sustained in the spleen and small intestine of weanling mice subjected to acute forms of malnutrition mimicking marasmus or incipient kwashiorkor [8]. Importantly, the latter outcome was reported in experimental systems shown repeatedly to induce a profound and disproportionate involution of T cell compartments including the systemically recirculating pool. These findings extend the data base that points to a regulated non-inflammatory form of immune competence to include tolerogenic cellular elements in addition to soluble mediators. Clearly this critical component of evidence requires a broader and deeper foundation including, in particular, assessment of the impact of malnutrition on the balance between inflammatory and regulatory functional capacities within the T cell compartment.

4. Conclusion

A research front designated “immunometabolism” has emerged from efforts to understand the inflammatory character of obesity and its associated chronic pathologies including type 2 diabetes and cardiovascular disease [55]. This new field reflects a realization that a mature and scholarly understanding of immune defences centers them within a systemic network of regulatory elements, both soluble and cellular, that govern the activities of all cells, tissues and physiological systems. The Tolerance Model offers similar conceptual sophistication, centered on the same basic principle, with respect to the large data base describing immune competence in acute malnutrition. As shown in Figure 3, the model is easily incorporated into the Malnutrition-Infection Cycle, thereby effecting a fundamental revision of this classic and foundational concept.

The Tolerance Model centers on a regulated, non-inflammatory immunological set-point specific to acute malnutrition. Importantly, the model neither invokes loss of control over components of immune competence such as cell-mediated inflammatory immunity nor suggests that any components of immune function might escape reform. Rather, it is proposed that malnutrition-associated immune defences remain universally subject to regulation and fine-tuning and that the redefined set-point of immune competence has its origins in an endocrine- and cytokine-mediated metabolic response that re-shapes all physiological functions. A nascent form of this proposition can be found occasionally in early literature pertaining to immune depression in pediatric malnutrition [e.g., 56], but the concept has never been developed sufficiently to support a paradigm shift.

Regulation is costly in metabolic terms and the Tolerance Model assumes this cost in the face of limited supplies of substrates and energy. However, unlike a biologically trivial disintegrative process leading to loss of control, a regulated phenomenon can respond to management intervention. Hence, the Tolerance Model provides a basis for optimism in an otherwise bleak clinical setting. More than a decade ago, immune competence was identified as an under-appreciated factor in the management of childhood malnutrition [57]. Pursuit of the implications of the Tolerance Model can reasonably be expected to yield clinical benefits in relation to the infection-related sequelae of acute protein and energy deficiencies. It is recognized that no adaptive attempt can be sustained indefinitely in the face of negative nitrogen and energy balance and, therefore, all aspects of immune competence must ultimately succumb to disintegrative loss as a consequence of unabated wasting disease. However, the Tolerance Model addresses a period of time, extending into the advanced stages of weight loss, during which immunological regulation evidently remains intact. From a clinical perspective, this represents a previously unrecognized window of opportunity to stabilize perhaps even the most debilitated patients. At present the Model centers on the pre-pubescent stage of life, but a small evidence base pertaining to hormonal interventions (32, 33, 43) and the generation of regulatory T cells (54) provides some basis for including adolescent and adult stages of development. In addition, there exists no *a priori* reason to exclude secondary forms of malnutrition from the Model, and this clinically significant possibility also deserves research attention.

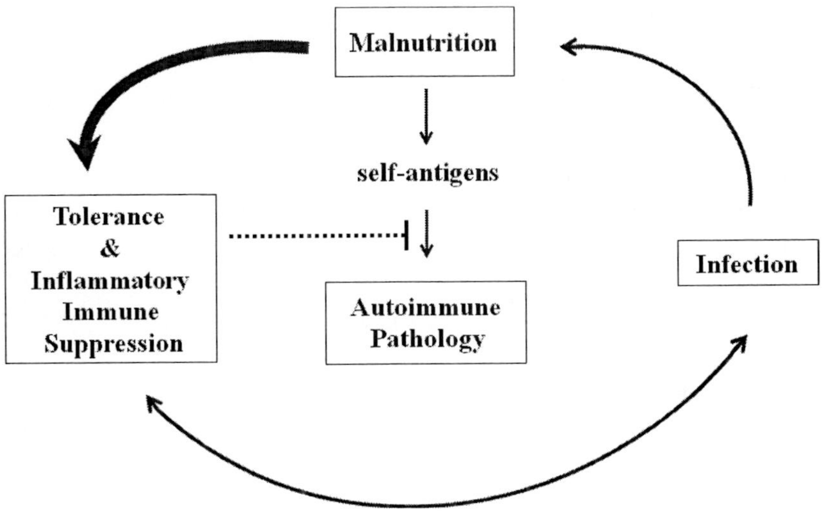

Figure 3. The classic Malnutrition-Infection Cycle depicted for acute deficits of protein and energy and modified to incorporate the Tolerance Model. The bolded arrow highlights the portion of the cycle governed by anti-inflammatory hormones and cytokines, e.g. glucocorticoids, TGF-β and IL-10. A bidirectional connection links infection and immune competence because many infections that are aggravated by malnutrition also reduce inflammatory capabilities.

Acknowledgments

Financial support received from the Natural Sciences and Engineering Research Council of Canada, a Discovery Grant to BW and a postdoctoral fellowship to JMM, is gratefully acknowledged.

References

[1] Collins, S. Treating severe acute malnutrition seriously. *Arch. Dis. Child.*, 2007, 92, 453-461.

[2] Pelletier, DL. The relationship between child anthro-pometry and mortality in developing countries: implications for policy, programs and future research. *J. Nutr.*, 1994, 124, 2047S-2081S.

[3] Woodward, B. The effect of protein-energy malnutrition on immune competence. In: *Suskind RM, Tontisirin K editors. Nutrition, Immunity, and Infection in Infants and Children.* Philadelphia: Vevey/Lippincott Williams and Wilkins; 2001; pp. 89-116.

[4] Botran, M; Lopez-Herce, J; Mencia, S; Urbano, J; Solana, MJ; Garcia, A; Carrillo, A. Relationship between energy expenditure, nutritional status and clinical severity before starting enteral nutrition in critically ill children. *Brit. J. Nutr.*, 2011, 105, 731-737.

[5] Hillyer, L; Dao, B; Niemiec, P; Lee, S; Doidge, M; Bemben, I; Neyestani, T; Woodward, B. Elevated bioactivity of the tolerogenic cytokines, interleukin-10 and transforming growth factor-β, in the blood of acutely malnourished weanling mice. *Exp. Biol. Med.*, 2006, 231, 1439-1447.

[6] Monk, JM; Woodward, B. Elevated blood interleukin-10 levels and undiminished systemic interleukin-10 production rate prevail throughout acute protein-energy malnutrition in the weanling mouse. *Cytokine,* 2009, 47, 126-131.

[7] Monk, JM; Woodward, B. The blood level of transforming growth factor-beta rises in the early stages of acute protein and energy deficit in the weanling mouse. *Brit. J. Nutr.*, 2010, 103, 886-889.

[8] Monk, JM; Richard, CL; Woodward, B. A non-inflammatory form of immune competence prevails in acute pre-pubescent malnutrition: new evidence based on critical mRNA transcripts in the mouse. *Brit. J. Nutr.*, in press.

[9] Monk, JM; Steevels, TAM; Hillyer, LM; Woodward, B. Constitutive, but not challenge-induced, interleukin-10 production is robust in acute pre-pubescent protein and energy deficits: New support for the tolerance hypothesis of malnutrition-associated immune depression based on cytokine production in vivo. *Int. J. Environ. Res. Public Health*, 2011, 8, 117-135.

[10] Dabadghao, P; Bhatia, E; Bhatia, V; Jayaraj, K; Colman, PG. Islet-cell antibodies in malnutrition-related diabetes mellitus in North India. *Diabetes Res. Clin. Prac.*, 1996, 34, 73-78.

[11] Unnikrishnan, AG; Singh, SK; Sanjeevi, CB. Prevalence of GAD65 antibodies in lean subjects with type 2 diabetes. *Ann. N Y Acad. Sci.,* 2004, 1037: 118-121.

[12] Woodward, B; Filteau, SM. Immunoenhancement in wasting protein-energy malnutrition: Assessment of present information and proposal of a new concept. *Adv. Nutr. Res.,* 1990, 8, 11-34.

[13] Matarese, G; La Cava, A; Sanna, V; Lord, GM; Lechler, RI; Fontana, S; Zappacosta, S. Balancing susceptibility to infection and autoimmunity: a role for leptin? *Trends Immunol*, 2002, 23, 182-87.

[14] Mestecky, J; Russell, MW; Elson, CO. Intestinal IgA: novel views on its function in defence of the largest mucosal surface. *Gut.,* 1999, 44, 2-5.

[15] Karagiannidis, C; Akdis, M; Holopainen, P; Woolley, NJ; Hense, G; Ruckert, B; Mantel, P-Y; Menz, G; Akdis, CA; Blaser, K; Schmidt-Weber, CB. Glucocorticoids upregulate FOXP3 expression and regulatory T cells in asthma. *J. Allergy Clin. Immunol.*, 2004, 114, 1425-1433.

[16] Li, MO; Falvell, RA. Contextual regulation of inflammation: a duet by transforming growth factor-β and interleukin-10. *Immunity*, 2008, 28, 468-476.

[17] Vignali, DAA; Collison, LW; Workman, CJ. How regulatory T cells work. *Nat. Rev. Immunol.*, 2008, 8, 523-532.

[18] Pugliese, MT. Endocrine function adaptations in undernutrition. *World Rev. Nutr. Dietet.,* 1990, 62, 186-211.

[19] Monk, JM; Makinen; Shrum, B; Woodward, B. Blood corticosterone concentration reaches critical illness levels early during acute malnutrition in the weanling mouse. *Exp. Biol. Med.*, 2006, 231, 264-268.

[20] Dai, G; McMurray, DN. Altered cytokine production and impaired antimycobacterial immunity in protein-malnourished guinea pigs. *Infec. Immun.,* 1998, 66, 3562-3568.

[21] Hillyer, LM; Maliwichi, HE; Woodward, B. Blood serum interferon-γ bioactivity is low in weanling mice subjected to acute deficits of energy or both protein and energy. *Brit. J. Nutr.*, 2007, 97, 528-534.

[22] Bienvenu, JAD; Monneret, G; Gutowski, MCl; Fabien, N. Cytokine assays in human sera and tissues. *Toxicol.*, 1998, 129, 55-61.

[23] Verbon, A; Juffermans, N; van Deventer, SJH; Speelman, P; van Deutekom, H; van der Pol, T. Serum concentrations of cytokines in patients with active tuberculosis (TB) and after treatment. *Clin. Exp. Immunol.,* 1999, 115, 110-113.

[24] Straus, DS; Burke, EJ; Marten, NW. Induction of insulin-like growth factor binding protein-1 gene expression in liver of protein-restricted rats and in rat hepatoma cells limited for a single amino acid. *Endocrinology,* 1993, 132, 1090-1100.

[25] Straus, DS; Marten, NW; Hayden, JM; Burke, EJ. Protein restriction specifically decreases the abundance of serum albumin and transthyretin nuclear transcripts in rat liver. *J. Nutr.*, 1994, 124, 1041-51.

[26] Mayatepek, E; Becker, K; Gana, L; Hoffmann, GF; Leichsenring, M. Leukotrienes in the pathophysiology of kwashiorkor. *Lancet,* 1993, 342, 958-960.

[27] Mayes, PA. Metabolism of unsaturated fatty acids and eicosanoids. In: Murray RK, Granner DK, Mayes PA, Rodwell VW editors. *Harper's Biochemistry (22nd edition).* San Mateo, CA: Appleton and Lange; 1990; pp. 218-225.

[28] Pace-Asciak, CR; Klein, J; Spielberg, SP. Human genetic defect in leukotriene C4 synthesis. *Biochem. Biophys. Res. Commun.*, 1986, 140, 857-860.

[29] Ingenbleek, Y. Thyroid dysfunction in protein-calorie malnutrition. *Nutr. Rev.,* 1986, 44, 253-263.

[30] Soliman, AT; El Zalabani, MM; Salama, M; Ansari, BM. Serum leptin concentrations during severe protein-energy malnutrition: Correlation with growth parameters and endocrine function. *Metabolism*, 2000, 49, 819-825.

[31] Barnes, PJ. Anti-inflammatory actions of glucocorticoids: molecular mechanisms. *Clin. Sci.*, 1998, 94, 557-572.

[32] Hill, ADK; Naama, HA; Gallagher, HJ; Shou, J; Calvano, SE; Daly, J. Glucocorticoids mediate macrophage dysfunction in protein calorie malnutrition. *Surgery*, 1995, 118, 130-137.

[33] Hill, ADK; Naama, H; Shou, J; Calvano, SE; Daly, JM. Antimicrobial effects of granulocyte-macrophage colony-stimulating factor in protein-energy malnutrition. *Arch. Surg.*, 1995, 130, 1273-1278.

[34] Fabris, N; Mocchegiani, E; Provinciali, M. Pituitary-thyroid axis and immune system: A reciprocal neuroendocrine-immune interaction. *Horm. Res.*, 1995, 43, 29-38.

[35] Kruger, TE. Immunomodulation of peripheral lymphocytes by hormones of the hypothalamus-pituitary-thyroid axis. *Adv. Neuroimmunol.*, 1996, 6, 387-395.

[36] Barlow, JW; De Nayer, P. Characterization of thyroid hormone receptors in human IM-9 lymphocytes. *Acta Endocrinol. (Copenh),* 1988, 117, 327-332.

[37] Mascanfroni, I; Montesinos, MM; Susperreguy, S; Cervi, L; Ilarregui, JM; Ramseyer, VD; Masini-Rapiso, AM; Targovnik, HM; Rabinovich,

GA; Pellizas, CG. Control of dendritic cell maturation and function by triiodothyronine. *FASEB J.,* 2008, 22, 1032-1042.

[38] Muller, MJ; Leymann, J; von zur Muhlen, A. Direct thermic effect of 3,5,3′-triiodothyronine: Microcalorimetric measurements of heat production in cultured mitogen-stimulated human T-lymphocytes. *Endocrine. J.,* 1994, 2, 343-348.

[39] Filteau, SM; Perry, KJ; Woodward, B. Triiodothyronine improves the primary antibody response to sheep red blood cells in severely undernourished weanling mice. *Proc. Soc. Exp. Biol. Med.*, 1987, 185, 427-433.

[40] Perry, KJ; Filteau, SM; Woodward, B. Dissociation of immune capacity from nutritional status by triiodothyronine supplements in severe protein deficiency. *FASEB J.*, 1988, 2, 2609-2612.

[41] Woods, JW; Woodward, BD. Enhancement of primary systemic acquired immunity by exogenous triiodothyronine in wasted, protein-energy malnourished weanling mice. *J. Nutr.*, 1991, 121, 1425-1432.

[42] Woods, JW; Woodward, B. Immunorestorative effect of triiodothyronine supplementation on the primary antibody response to sheep red blood cells following development of immunodepression in protein-energy malnourished weanling mice. *J. Nutr. Immunol.*, 1994, 3, 3-12.

[43] Lord, GM; Matarese, G; Howard, JK; Baker, RJ; Bloom, SR; Lechler, RI. Leptin modulates the T-cell immune response and reverses starvation-induced immunosuppression. *Nature*, 1998, 394, 897-901.

[44] Faggioni, R; Feingold, KR; Grunfeld, C. Leptin regulation of the immune response and the immunodeficiency of malnutrition. *FASEB J.,* 2001, 15, 2565-2571.

[45] Merad, M; Manz, MG. Dendritic cell homeostasis. *Blood*, 2009, 113, 3418 – 3427.

[46] Hillyer, LM. *Response of the acutely malnourished weanling mouse to exogenous murine FMS-like tyrosine kinase 3 ligand.* MSc Thesis, University of Guelph, Ontario, Canada; 2008.

[47] Kedl, RM; Rees, WA; Hildeman, DA; Schaefer, B; Mitchell, T; Kappler, J; Marrack, P. T cells compete for access to antigen-bearing antigen-presenting cells. *J. Exp. Med.*, 2000, 192, 1105-1113.

[48] Gonzalez-Martinez, H; Rodriguez, L; Najera, O; Cruz, D; Miliar, A; Dominguez, A; Sanchez, F; Graniel, J; Gonzalez-Torres, MC. Expression of cytokine mRNA in lymphocytes of malnourished children. *J. Clin. Immunol.,* 2008, 28, 593-599.

[49] Finkelman, FD; Morris, S; Orekhova, T; Orekhova, T; Sehy, D. The in vivo cytokine capture assay for measurement of cytokine production in the mouse. In: Coligan JE, Bierer BE, Margulies DH, Shevach EM, Strober W editors. *Current protocols in immunology* (Unit 6.28). New York, NY: John Wiley and Sons, Inc; 2003; pp. 1-10.
[50] Steevels, TAM; Hillyer, LM; Monk, JM; Fisher, ME; Woodward, BD. Effector/memory T cells of the weanling mouse exhibit type 2 cytokine polarization in vitro and in vivo in the advanced stages of acute energy deficit. *J. Nutr. Biochem.*, 2010, 21, 504-511.
[51] Fernandez-Botran, R; Vitetta, ES. Evidence that natural murine soluble interleukin 4 receptors may act as transport proteins. *J. Exp. Med.*, 1991, 174, 673-681.
[52] Bendtzen, K; Svenson, M; Jonsson, V; Hippe, E. Autoantibodies to cytokines – friends or foes? *Immunol. Today*, 1990, 11, 167-169.
[53] Sakaguchi, S; Ono, M; Setoguchi, R; Yagi, H; Hori, S; Fehervari, Z; Shimizu, J; Takahashi, T; Nomura, T. Foxp3+ CD25+ CD4+ natural regulatory T cells in dominant self-tolerance and autoimmune disease. *Immunol. Rev.*, 2006, 212, 8-27.
[54] Procaccini, C; De Rosa, V; Galgani, M; Abanni, L; Cali, G; Porcellini, A; Carbone, F; Fontana, S; Horvath, TL; La Cava, A; Matarese, G. An oscillatory switch in mTOR kinase activity sets regulatory T cell responsiveness. *Immunity,* 2010, 33, 929-941.
[55] Mathis, D; Shoelson, SE. Immunometabolism: an emerging frontier. *Nature Rev. Immunol.,* 2011, 11, 81-83.
[56] Schonland, MM; Shanley, BC; Loening, WEK; Parent, MA; Coovadia, HM. Plasma cortisol and immunosuppression in protein-calorie malnutrition. *Lancet*, 1972, ii, 435-436.
[57] Chevalier, P; Sevilla, R; Sejas, E; Zalles, L; Belmonte, G; Parent, G. Immune recovery of malnourished childrentakes longer than nutritional recovery: implications for treatment and discharge. *J. Trop. Pediatr.,* 1998, 44, 304-307.

Reviewed by Dr. Carla Taylor, Department of Human Nutritional Sciences, University of Manitoba, Winnipeg, Canada

In: Malnutrition: Risk Factors ...
Editor: J.B. Knudsen

ISBN: 978-1-62100-351-9

Chapter 5

Genotoxic Effects of Malnutrition and Infections in Argentinean Children

Gisel Padula[1,2,3] ***and Analía Seoane***[1,3]
[1]IGEVET, (Instituto de Genética Veterinaria), UNLP-CONICET, La Plata, Argentina
[2]Facultad de Ciencias Naturales y Museo, Universidad Nacional de La Plata, Argentina
[3]CONICET (Consejo Nacional de Investigaciones Científicas y Técnicas), Argentina

Abstract

The purpose of this study was to evaluate the relationship between malnutrition, bacterial infections and citogenetic damage. In order to obtain the frequencies of structural chromosomal aberrations (SCAs) in peripheral blood lymphocytes, we sample malnourished and eutrophic children with and without bacterial infections. Fifty infants concurrent to the Hospital Interzonal de Agudos y Crónicos Dr. Alejandro Korn, La Plata, Argentina were included in this study; 14 malnourished and non-infected (MN), 11 malnourished and infected (MI), 18 eutrophic and non-infected (EN) and 7 eutrophic and infected (EI). Children aged 1-60 months. Anthropometric and clinic evaluation were performed to assess nutritional condition. Before blood collection, we interviewed each individual's parent to complete a semi structural survey specifying age, dietary habits, bacterial diseases; previous exposure to diagnostic x-rays; and use of therapeutic drugs. After 48 hours, 100 cultured lymphocytes were analyzed per individual. Statistical analysis was performed by the Epi Info 6.0, through the Pearson $\chi 2$ Test ($p<0.05$). No significant differences were found in total SCA frequency between MN and MI (14.2% vs. 15.1%). In MN children the total SCA frequency was four times higher than that of EI ones (14.2% vs. 3.33% $p<0.001$), and eight times higher than that of EN ones (14.2 vs. 1.8 <0.001). As well, in MI children the total SCA frequency was five times higher than that of EI ones (15.1% vs. 3.33% $p<0.001$) and eight times higher than that of EN ones (15.1 vs. 1.8 <0.001). Meanwhile the total SCA frequency was two times greater in EI than in EN children (3.33% vs. 1.88% $p<0.05$). Results presented here showed an increase frequency of SCA not only in relation with malnutrition but also with the presence of bacterial infections. However the effect of malnutrition was more important than the other. It is difficult to discern whether structural chromosome aberrations are due to malnutrition per se, bacterial or viral infections, or all of these factors acting on malnourished tissues. DNA damage could be attributed to several reasons: severe deficiency of essential nutrients (i.e. zinc, iron, and vitamin A) required in the synthesis of DNA maintenances factors; decline of repair mechanisms; and/or the absence of specific substances needed to protect the cell against oxidative DNA damage. In conclusion, mutagenic agents cause chromosomal changes more easily in an altered environment.

Keywords: Primary Protein Energy Malnutrition, Bacterial Infections, Structural Chromosome Aberrations, Children

INTRODUCTION

Growth was defined as a process resulting from the continuous and complex interaction of inheritance and environment (Tanner, 1986). In developed countries, genetic factors are responsible of most of growth retardations. On the contrary, in developing countries, nutritional deficit is frequently the cause of growth retardations. Malnutrition occurs when there is a cellular imbalance between the supply of nutrients and energy and the body's demand for them to ensure growth, maintenance, and specific functions (Waterlow, 1996). In this sense the term protein-energy malnutrition applies to a group of related disorders that develop in children and adults whose consumption of protein and energy (measured by calories) is insufficient to satisfy the body's nutritional needs (primary PEM). PEM may also occur in persons who are unable to absorb vital nutrients or convert them to energy essential for healthy tissue formation and organ function (secondary PEM) (Más Vida, 2002; Padula et al., 2009). PEM results from food insufficiency as well as from poor social and economic conditions, children with PEM lose their resistance to infectious diseases due to immune system disorders (Dulger et al., 2002).

In addition, malnutrition has been associated with high levels of DNA damage as a result of various factors, including the possibility that the cells of malnourished children are more susceptible to environmental damage (Gonzalez et al., 2002; Padula et al ., 2004; Padula et al., 2009). In this regard, some authors (Betancourt et al., 1995; Ortiz et al., 1997; Gonzalez et al. 2002a and b) reported an increase in DNA damage in malnourished children with bacterial infections with respect to eutrophic children with bacterial infections.

The purpose of this chapter was to evaluate the relationship between malnutrition, bacterial infections and citogenetic damage, in children peripheral blood lymphocytes.

Materials and Methods

Experimental Procedure

Fifty primary malnourished infants concurrent to the Consultorio del Niño Sano of the Hospital Interzonal de Agudos y Crónicos Dr. Alejandro Korn, La Plata, Argentina were included in this analysis; 14 malnourished and non-infected (MN), 11 malnourished and infected (MI) (with gastrointestinal or respiratory bacterial infections), 18 eutrophic and non-infected (EN) and 7 eutrophic and infected (EI). Children were aged 1 to 60 months. Anthropometric and clinic evaluation were performed to assess nutritional condition. Before blood collection, we interviewed each individual's parent to complete a semi structural survey specifying age, dietary habits, bacterial diseases; previous exposure to diagnostic x-rays; and use of therapeutic drugs for 1 month before the study. Also, children with anemia or signs of vitamin deficiency were not included in this study. Specific written information about the aims of the study was provided to all participants.Written informed consent was obtained from the participants' parents (Ley Provincial N° 11044).

Cytogenetic Analysis

Heparinized venous blood samples were used to obtain lymphocytes from the participants and set up 2 replicate cultures, using 1 ml total blood in 9 ml RPMI 1640 medium (Gibco-Invitrogen Buenos Aires, Argentina) containing 1% phytohemagglutinin (Gibco-Invitrogen), 100 IU penicillin, and 100 μg/ml streptomycin (Sigma, St. Louis, MO). The cultures were incubated at 37°C and 5% CO^2 for 48 hours. Two hours before harvesting, colchicine was added at a final concentration of 0.1 g/ml. The cells were harvested by centrifugation. Metaphases were obtained by routine protocols and stained with 5% Giemsa, (Spectrum Chemicals, Gardena, CA). Structural chromosome aberrations were scored in 100 metaphases per individual by using a blind analysis: one investigator numerically identified the samples, and another scored the aberrations. Only metaphases with 46 chromosomes were considered. The identification of SCA was carried out by following the criteria recommended by Archer and coworkers (1981) and the World Health Organization (1985). Mitotic Index (MI) was calculated. Statistical analysis was performed using the Epi Dat 3.0 (OPS-OMS, 2003), through «Test de Diferencias entre dos proporciones muestrales». The differences were considered significant if the probability values were less than .05.

Anthropometric Evaluation

Height (H), weight (W), mid upper arm circumference (MUAC), triceps (TS) and subscapular skinfold (SS) were measured. The height for age index (H//A), the weight for age index (W//A), the weight for height index (W//H), the mid upper arm circumference for age index (MUAC//A), the triceps skinfold for age index (TS//A) and the subscapular skinfold for age index (SS//A) were calculated. Variables were introduced into the EpiInfo 6.04 program (CDC-OMS, 2001) and transformed into z-scores, using the NCHS anthropometric standards as reference (1977). A z-score of less than –1.1 was the cut-off point to determine the prevalence of stunting, underweight and wasting respectively. Malnutrition degrees were established according to Torun and Chew (1994). For children younger than 2 years, the H//A and W//A, stunting and underweight indicators, were used. H//A and W//H, stunting and wasting indicators modified from Waterlow (1976), were applied for the others. These classification include the following classes: 1) normal: W//H adequate with normal stature, 2) stunting: W//H adequate with low stature, 3) wasting: W//H low with normal stature, 4) stunting and wasting: W//H low with low stature.

RESULTS

The anthropometric classification of the malnourished children is shown in Tables 1 and 2. Table 3 shows the results of cytogenetic analysis. No significant differences were found in total SCA frequency between MN and MI (14.2% vs. 15.1%). In MN children the total SCA frequency was four times higher than that of EI ones (14.2% vs. 3.33% $p<0.001$), and eight times higher than that of EN ones (14.2 vs. 1.8 <0.001). As well, in MI children the total SCA frequency was five times higher than that of EI ones (15.1% vs. 3.33% $p<0.001$) and eight times higher than that of EN ones (15.1 vs. 1.8 <0.001). Meanwhile the total SCA frequency was two times greater in EI than in EN children (3.33% vs. 1.88% $p<0.05$).

Table 1. Anthropometric evaluation of malnourished children using H//A, W//A, W//H indexes

	<2 y old					>2 y old							
	Underweight		Underweight and Stunting			Wasting		Wasting and Stunting			Stunting	
Sex	D1	D2	D1	D2	D3	D1	D2	D1	D2	D3	D1	D2
Female	1	1	1	1	0	1	1	0	1	0	0	0
Male	0	0	1	1	0	0	0	0	0	1	0	1
Total	1	1	2	2	0	1	1	0	1	1	o	1

D1: degree 1; D2: degree 2; D3: degree 3.

Table 2. Anthropometric evaluation of malnourished children using mid upper arm circumference for age index (MUAC//A), triceps skinfold for age index (TS//A) and subscapular skinfold for age index (SS//A)

	MUAC//A			TS//A			SS//A		
Sex	E	LR	VLR	E	LR	VLR	E	LR	VLR
Female	0	1	6	1	6	0	1	4	2
Male	0	0	4	1	1	2	1	0	3
Total	0	1	10	2	7	2	2	4	5

E: euthrophic; LR: low reserve; VLR: very low reserve.

Table 3. Structural chromosome aberrations (SCA) in malnourished and non-infected (MN), malnourished and infected (MI), eutrophic and non-infected (EN) and eutrophic and infected (EI) children

SCA	MN		MI		EN		EI	
	Absolute	Percentage	Absolute	Percentage	Absolute	Percentage	Absolute	Percentage
Chtg	49	3.83	45	4.41	9	0.52	8	1.33
Chrg	14	1.09	8	0.78	4	0.23	0	0
Chtb	48	3.75	35	3.43	4	0.23	3	0.5
Chrb	6	0.47	4	0.39	0	0	1	0.17
Ace	36	2.81	21	2.06	3	0.17	3	0.5
Dic	4	0.31	5	0.49	0	0	0	0
r	0	0	0	0	0	0	0	0
Tas	25	1.95	36	3.53	11	0.64	5	0.83
Total SCA	182	14.2	154	15.1	31	1.8	20	3.33
Total Cells	1280	85.8	1020	84.9	1720	98.2	600	96.67

chtg: monochromatid gaps; chrg: isochromatid gaps; chtb: monochromatid breaks; chrb: isochromatid breaks; ace: fragments; dic: dicentric chromosomes; r: rings; tas: telomeric associations.

When detailed analysis was carried out, MN children showed similar frequencies of gaps, breaks, fragments and dicentric chromosomes than MI, only telomeric associatios was significantly lower in MN ($p<0.05$). On the other hand, MN children showed higher percentages of gaps, breaks, fragments, dicentric chromosomes and telomeric associations than EI and EN. These differences were significant for gaps ($p<0.01$), monochromatid breaks ($p<0.001$), fragments ($p<0.05$) and telomeric associations ($p<0.01$, only MN vs. EN) frequencies. Comparable results were found for MI vs. EI and EN. In addition, EI children showed higher rates of gaps, breaks, fragments and telomeric associations in compare to EN ones.

Children exposition to potential genotoxic agents, just as medication, radiation, pesticides and industrial residues, showed no significant differences between groups.

Discussion

Our results showed an increase frequency of SCA not only in relation with malnutrition but also with the presence of bacterial infections. Nevertheles, malnutrition induced damage was higher than the other. In the same way, others authors (Armendares et al., 1971; Khouri y McLaren, 1973; Betancourt et al., 1974; Upadhyaya et al., 1975a y b; Ortiz et al., 1997; Murthy et al., 1980; Betancourt et al., 1995), observed increase DNA damage in healthy infected versus healthy non-infected children and in malnourished infected versus healthy infected children. Results reported by Gonzalez and colleagues (2002a and b), agree with those above mentioned and confirmed that malnutrition and severe infections are two factors clearly associated with DNA damage increase.

In addition, Gonzalez and coworkers (2002b) observed significant increments of DNA damage assessed by comet assay in malnourished infected versus healthy infected children under medical treatment, suggesting that malnutrition enhance drug susceptibility inducing DNA damage. In malnutrition, it is likely to be impaired drug metabolism alterations because of the delay in absorption, reducing linkage protein, changes in the distribution volume, redox changes in the liver and reducing of the renal clearance. Krishnaswamy (1989) has reported that gentamicin half life is 25% higher and depuration 50% lower in malnourished versus eutrophic children. Drugs plasma concentrations were higher in malnutrition than in healthy state (Waterlow, 1996). It must be considered that energy and amino acids are requirements for proper protein synthesis process. In children fed protein-low diets, protein synthesis decreases by 25% (Jackson et al., 1983). Malnutrition means a decrease in the availability of energy or essential amino acids and it can cause a decrease in protein synthesis affecting the production of enzymes required for DNA repair. Induced DNA lesions are repaired efficiently by the cellular repair processes. This process involves many steps and interference with any of them will lead to negative biological effects, including chromosome aberrations (Natarajan, 2002). González and coworkers (2002) found a reduction in the repair ability in lymphocytes of malnourished children. The damage observed in malnourished children could be due to the deficiency of several essential nutrients required to protein synthesis that are associated with DNA integrity, impaired DNA repair mechanisms, and/or to the unavailability of molecules necessary to protect the cells against DNA oxidative damage. A cell with diminished ability to repair is likely to mutate more easily triggering processes of mutagenesis, carcinogenesis, teratogenesis, early senescence or even apoptosis (Zeiger and Tennant, 1986; Hagmar et al., 1998; Natarajan, 2002). For the foregoing, it is difficult to discern whether structural chromosome aberrations are due to malnutrition per se, bacterial and viral infections, antibiotics or all of these factors acting on malnourished tissues. Chromosomal damage could be attributed to several factors: a severe deficiency of essential nutrients and energy required for the synthesis of DNA maintenance factors; deterioration of repair mechanisms allowing the persistence of an abnormally high number of SCA; and/or the lack of specific factors that are needed to protect the cell against oxidative DNA damage. Further studies will be necessary involving a large number of patients to address the relationship between levels of DNA damage and specific kinds of infection, drug treatments, and the type and severity of malnutrition.

Conclusions

Severe infection would be associated with chromosomal damage and would have a more important effect in malnourished children. This fact could be explained by the alteration of DNA repair mechanisms.

References

Albertini RJ, Anderson D, Douglas GR, Hagmar L, Hemminki K, Merlo F, Natarajan AT, Norppa H, Shuker DE, Tice R, Waters MD, Aitio A (2000). IPCS guidelines for the monitoring of genotoxic effects of carcinogens in humans. International Programme on Chemical Safety. *Mutat. Res.* 463:111-72.

Archer PG, Bender M, Bloom AD, Brewen JG, Carrano AV, Preston RJ. Guidelines for cytogenetic studies in mutagen-exposed human populations. In: Bloom AD, ed. Guidelines for Studies on Human Populations Exposed to Mutagenic and Reproductive Hazards. *White Plains,* NY: March of Dimes Birth Defects Foundation; 1981:1–35.

Armendares S, Salamanca F y Frenk S (1971). Chromosome abnormalities in severe protein calorie malnutrition. *Nature* 232: 271-273.

Betancourt M, Ortíz R, González C, Pérez P, Cortés L, Rodríguez L, Villasenor L (1995). Assessment of DNA damage in leukocytes from infected and malnourished children by single cell gel electrophoresis/ comet assay. *Mutat. Res.* 331(1):65-77.

Carrano AV, Natarajan AT (1988). International Commission for Protection Against Environmental Mutagens and Carcinogens. ICPEMC publication no. 14. Considerations for population monitoring using cytogenetic techniques. *Mutat. Res.* 204:379-406.

Dulger H, Arik M, Sekeroglu MR, Tarakcioglu M, Noyan T, Cesur Y, Balahoroglu R (2002). Pro-inflammatory cytokines in Turkish children with protein-energy malnutrition. *Mediators Inflamm.* 11(6):363-365.

Epi Info. CDC / OMS. Procesador de texto, Base de datos y Estadística, para la Salud Pública. *Versión* 6.04d. 2001.

Epidat. OPS / OMS. Programa para análisis epidemiológico de datos tabulados. Versión 3.0. *Xunta de Galicia.* 2003.

González C, Najera O, Cortes E, Toledo G, Lopez L, Betancourt M, Ortiz R (2002b). Susceptibility to DNA damage induced by antibiotics in lymphocytes from malnourished children. *Teratog. Carcinog. Mutagen.* 22(2):147-158.

González C, Najera O, Cortés E, Toledo G, López L, Betancourt M, Ortíz R (2002a). Hydrogen peroxide-induced DNA damage and DNA repair in lymphocytes from malnourished children, *Environ. Mol. Mutagen.* 39(1):33-42.

Guide to short-term tests for detecting mutagenic, carcinogenic chemicals. In: Environmental Health Criteria 51. Geneva, Switzerland. *World Health Organization;* 1985:57–67.

Hagmar L, Bonassi S, Stromberg U, Brogger A, Knudsen LE, Norppa H, Reuterwall C (1998). Chromosomal aberrations in lymphocytes predict cancer: a report from the European Study Group on Cytogenetic Biomarkers and Health (ESCH), *Cancer Res.* 58: 4117-4121.

International System for Human Citogenetic Nomenclature (1995). Recommendations of the International Standing Committee on Human Cytogenetic Nomenclature, *Memphis, Tenn., Mitelman* F (Ed.).

Jackson AA, Golden MHN (1983). Whole body protein turnover and nitrogen balance in young children at intakes of protein and energy in the region of maintenance. *Human Nutrition: Clinical Nutrition* 37C: 433-446.

Khouri FP, McLaren DS (1973). Cytogenetic studies in protein-calorie malnutrition. *Am. J. Hum. Genet.* 25: 465-470.

Krishnaswamy K (1989). Drug metabolism and pharmacokinetics in malnourished children. *Clinical Pharmacokinetics* 17 (1): 68-88.

Murthy PB, Bhaskaram P, Srikantia SG (1980). Sister chromatid exchanges in protein-energy malnutrition. *Hum. Genet.* 55: 404-406.

Natarajan AT (2002). Chromosome aberrations: past, present and future. *Mutat. Res.* 504: 3-16.

NCHS/OMS. Growth curves for children. Birth- 18 years. *Vital and Health Statistics.* US Department of Health, Education, and Welfare. Public Health Service. 1977. Series 11:165.

Ortiz R, Cortes L, Gonzalez C, Lopez L, Perez P, Cortes E, Betancourt M (1997). Analysis of mitomycin C-induced micronuclei in lymphocytes from malnourished infected children. *Environ. Mol. Mutagen.* 30(4): 363-370.

Padula G, Salceda SA, Prozzi M, Fernández A, Seoane A (2004). Alteraciones Cromosómicas en niños con Malnutrición Proteico-Energética: resultados preliminares. *Ludovica Pediátrica.* Publicación Científica del Hospital Sor María Ludovica de La Plata. ISSN 1514-5654. Vol VI (2):43-50.

Programa Más Vida (2002). Guía Normativa sobre desnutrición. Tanner JM. El Hombre antes del Hombre. *El crecimiento físico desde la concepción hasta la madurez.* México: Fondo de Cultura Económica; 1986.

Terreros MC, De Luca JC, Dulout FN (1993). The effect of a Hypoproteic Diet and Ethano Consumption on the Yield of Chromosoma Damage Detected in Bone Marrow Cells o Mice. *J. Vet. Med. Sci.* 55 (2):191-194.

Torun B, Chew F (1994). Protein Energy Malnutrition. En: *Modern Nutrition in Health and disease.* Shils ME, Olson JA y Shike M (eds.). Lea and Febiger (editorial). 8 Edición. Vol 2.

Upadhyaya KC, Uerma IC, Ghai OP (1975) Chromosomal aberrations in protein-caloriemalnutrition. *Lancet* 2: 704.

Upadhyaya KC, Uerma IC,y Ghai OP (1975). Chromosome aberrations in protein-calorie malnutrition. *Indian Pediatr.* 12: 857-863.

Waterlow JC, Buzina R, Keller W, Lane JM, Nichman MZ, Tanner JM (1977). The presentation and use of the Weight and Height data for comparing the nutritional status of groups of children under the age of 10 years. *Bull. WHO* 55: 489.

Waterlow JC. Malnutrición proteico-energética. Organización Panamericana de la Salud. Organización Mundial de la Salud. *Publicación Científica* Nro. 555. Washington. D.C.; 1996.

Zeiger E, Tennant RW (1986). Mutagenesis, clastogenesis, carcinogenesis: expectations, correlations and relations. *Prog. Clin. Biol. Res.* 209:75-84.

In: Malnutrition: Risk Factors …
Editor: J.B. Knudsen
ISBN: 978-1-62100-351-9

Chapter 6

INFLUENCE OF NUTRITIONAL SUPPORT ON NUTRITIONAL AND MENTAL STATUS IN DEMENTIA PATIENTS WITH ALZHEIMER'S DISEASE: COMPARATIVE AND INTERVENTION STUDY

M. Navrátilová[1], J. Jarkovský[2], E. Češková[1], A. Vašků[3], B. Leonard[4] and L. Sobotka[5]

[1]Department of Psychiatry, Faculty of Medicine, Masaryk University, Brno, Czech Republic

[2]Institute of Biostatistics and Analyses, Faculty of Medicine and Faculty of Science, Masaryk University, Brno, Czech Republic

[3]Department of Pathological Physiology, Faculty of Medicine, Masaryk University, Brno, Czech Republic

[4]Pharmacology Department, National University of Ireland, Galway, Ireland

[5]Department of Metabolic Care and Gerontology, Faculty of Medicine, Charles University, Hradec Králové, Czech Republic

SUMMARY

Background: Alzheimer's disease (AD) is a degenerative disease of the central nervous system and its progression is often connected with a development of severe malnutrition. However, sufficient data on nutritional state and intervention regarding the progression of AD have not yet been available. The aims of our study were: a) to describe the relation between the state of mental function and nutritional status in patients with Alzheimer's disease and in those with dementia of vascular aetiology, b) to assess the relationship between nutritional support and the improvement, or the maintenance, of the patients' state of health.

Methods: 165 patients from 7 institutions throughout the Czech Republic were included in a two-year-study. Voluntary food intake was measured during the first year following which the patients with Alzheimer's disease were randomised into two groups. The study group received 600 kcal supplements to their regular diet whereas the control group continued on standard diet. The nutritional parameters using the Mini Nutritional Assessment (MNA), body weight, triceps skin fold and mental state Mini Mental State Examination (MMSE) and Clock Drawing Test were monitored every second month of the study period.

Findings: a) the nutritional status (MNA) was significantly worse in patients with Alzheimer's disease than in the patients with vascular dementia. The patients with Alzheimer's dementia who died had been suffering from severe malnutrition during the last three months of their lives. b) There was discovered a significant decline of the mental functions in Alzheimer's disease patients also suffered from malnutrition. Nutritional support significantly slowed down the deterioration of the mental functions of the AD patients.

Interpretation: Our study showed that patients with AD are more undernourished than patients suffering from the vascular type of dementia, in spite of similar voluntary energy intake. Nutritional intervention significantly decreased the progression of the deterioration of the AD patients′ mental functions as well as other complications. It is concluded, that dietary counselling and nutritional support in patients with AD is clinically important and reduces the impairment of mental functions.

Keywords: Alzheimer's disease; malnutrition; nutritional support, sipping, Mini Nutritional Assessment (MNA); Mini Mental State Examination (MMSE)

INTRODUCTION

Alzheimer's disease (AD) is a degenerative disease of the central nervous system, affecting at least 3% of the population worldwide. The progressive dementia in this disease was described by the German psychiatrist Alois Alzheimer's in his lecture in Tübingen already in 1906 [1]. The disease occurs most often after the 65th year of age, when the prevalence is 10%, but it can occur also in younger individuals. In persons of over 85 years of age the prevalence of AD is estimated to make more than 20% and in the Europe almost 6 million people suffer from this disease [2]. The course of the disease is characterized predominantly by a gradual loss of cognitive functions, increasing behavioural difficulties with a subsequent decrease of independence and dementia. Moreover, AD is regularly connected with a significant and gradual body weight loss.

It is known that about 40% of the AD patients lose 4% of their body weight a year; the loss of muscle mass is especially serious. The loss of muscle mass worsens the response to physiotherapy, increases the risk of infectious complications and the occurrence of bed sores [3, 4]. Loss of muscle mass can also lead to a gradual decline in the quality of life and considerably reduces the survival rate. A loss of body weight greater than 5% in a year is considered a bad prognostic indicator in AD patients [5]. On the other hand, an increase in body weight lowers the mortality rate in these patients [4]. According to our clinical experience it was shown that body weight loss is more pronounced in AD patients than in patients with dementia of vascular aetiology. In spite of this information, studies that assess long-term nutritional status in dementia patients are rare, those studies that determine the effect of nutritional support on the survival and psychological outcome of AD patients are still lacking.

Therefore our study was designed to:

1. Describe the nutritional status and voluntary food intake in patients with AD and in patients with dementia of vascular origin during a two years´ period, to observe their dynamics prospectively and to compare those two groups of patients.
2. To establish the effect of nutritional intervention on energy intake, survival rate and on the state of mental functions in the group of patients with AD.

Material and Methods

Patients

165 patients suffering from AD dementia or dementia of vascular origin were included in our study. They were institutionalised in seven nursing homes for the elderly throughout the Czech Republic and were monitored for three years with a median of 9 observations and a basic observation time every two months. In the patient group there were 100 with AD diagnosis and 65 with vascular dementia (VD). The characteristic of the patients is stated in Table 1.

Table 1. Characteristic of the study group

		AD	VD
No.		100	65
Male		19	13
Female		81	52
Age*	Mean	78.9	81.7
	Median	79.0	82.3
	Min	58.0	56.2
	Max	94.0	97.0
No. of deceased patients		62	49

AD – Alzheimer's disease, VD – Vascular dementia

Diagnosis

The diagnosis AD had been established by two independent psychiatrists (the local physician and the physician of the relevant institution) according to the ICD-10 [6]. Apart from the clinical examination, the diagnosis of dementia was confirmed by the MMSE and the diagnosis of vascular dementia was further confirmed by an examination using the Hachinski Ischaemia Score [7].

Study Design

The patients were divided into two groups according to the psychiatric examination mentioned above. After the start of the study, both groups (AD and VD) were compared regarding the psychological functions and nutritional status. Then a comparison of the dynamics of the mental and nutritional state was performed in the patients who survived and in those who had died (end of study) in both groups. The patients were monitored for one year without any nutritional supplementation.

After the first year of the study the AD patients were randomly divided into two groups. The first group received nutritional supplementation in the form of liquid polymeric enteral nutrition daily (Nutridrink multifiber, Nutricia, The Netherlands). This liquid formulation was supplied twice a day between lunch and dinner (at 2.00 p.m.) and before bedtime (at 9.00 p.m.) to prevent interference with normal food intake. The total daily amount of nutrients given to the supplemented group was 600 kcal/day (proteins 24g /day, carbohydrates 74 g/day, lipids 23 g day, fibres 9 g/day). The control group continued consuming ordinary food without nutritional supplements.

After the randomisation process, the groups were tested for comparability. No significant differences regarding the demographic characteristics (age, sex), or regarding the nutritional (MNA, skin fold) or mental state (MMSE, Clock Drawing Test) had been found between both groups.

Measurements

- The mental state of the patients was assessed once every 4 months using
  - Mini-mental state examination MMSE [8]
  - the Clock Drawing Test [9]
- The nutritional status and the risk of malnutrition occurrence were monitored with the help of
  - the body mass index (BMI) [10] once every 2 months (1325 recordings)
  - the skin fold thickness above the m.triceps brachii once every 2 months (1275 recordings)
  - the Mini nutritional assessment score (MNA) [11] once every 2 months (1325 recordings)
- The food intake was measured during 2 subsequent weekdays and once at a weekend every 2 months. The amount of the food consumed

was measured using the difference between the weight of the food that had been served and the weight of the food residue on the plate after eating (4605 records). The amounts of energy, proteins, carbohydrates and lipids were precisely calculated using the recipes with the help of food tables, using the computer programme Nutricom 2001 [12]. The mean value of the three-day records was calculated for each time period.

Statistical Analysis

The statistical analysis consists of two parts i) the patients were generally compared on behalf of their time range average, ii) the time ranges of the patients were aggregated by average into several time categories related towards the end of the monitoring or the decease of the patient due to the establishment of the analysis of the assessed parameters' trends. At the same time the patients' state at the beginning and at the end of the study were compared and a special analysis of the influence of the nutritional support was carried out.

Due to the nature of the data, non – parametric tests were used, namely the Mann Whitney test and the Kruskal Wallis ANOVA for the comparison of the groups and Spearman's correlation for the analysis of the relationship between the parameters. The comparison of the time categories was also performed using the Kruskal Wallis ANOVA, due to the different numbers of the patients assessed during the individual time spans of the monitoring. Wilcoxon's test for pair data was used only for the evaluation of the differences in the parameters between the beginning and the end of the study.

The two groups of patients (with and without nutritional support) were compared between the beginning of the study (first year) and the second part of the study (Kruskall-Wallis ANOVA). The frequency of occurrence of various events (decease etc.) in relation to the type of disease was analysed by the Fisher Exact Test.

The statistical analyses were carried out in the Statistic for Windows software. [13]

RESULTS

Nutritional Status and Outcome in AD and VD Patients

The VD patients were significantly older (age median 81.7 years, range 56-97 years) than the patients with AD (age median 78.9 years, range 58-94 years) (Mann Whitney U test, $p=0.016$). Three years mortality rate of AD patients (in the entire duration of the study) was significantly higher than that of the VD patients (75.4% vs. 59.0% respectively, Fisher exact test, $p=0.032$).

According to the MNA, in the group of patients with AD, 28% of the patients were at risk of severe malnutrition, 64% at risk of moderate malnutrition and only 8% were not at risk of malnutrition. In the group of patients with the vascular type of dementia 17% of the patients were suffering from severe malnutrition, 72% were moderately malnourished and 11% were without malnutrition. These differences between the groups were not statistically significant.

The BMI of up to 22 $kg.m^{-2}$ was recorded in 43.3% of the AD patients and in 25% of the patients with vascular dementia. The BMI was significantly lower in the AD patients than in the patients with vascular dementia (23.0 ± 3.6 vs. 25.5 ± 5.0 $kg.m^{-2}$ - $p<0.001$).

There was a trend to higher frequency of severe malnutrition (expressed as MNA) in AD patients (55%) than in the patients with vascular dementia (35.5%), during the last three months of life, however, this difference was not statistically significant (Fisher exact test, $p=0.161$).

The MNA score was strongly associated with the mortality rate of the patients, the deceased AD patients having had the lowest values of the score (Kruskal Wallis ANOVA, $p=0.02$, Figure 1). Patients with AD who died during the study had the lowest values of MMSE (Kruskal Wallis ANOVA, $p<0.001$, Figure 2). Statistically significant differences were found also when comparing the skin fold thickness and the BMI between the groups, using the combination of the diagnosis and the death rate of the patients (Figure 3, 4).

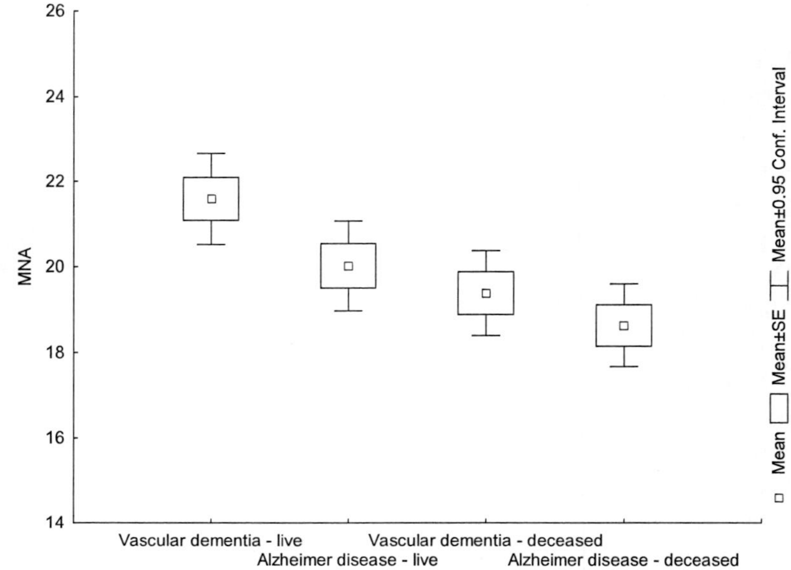

Figure 1. MNA score within groups of patients defined by their diagnosis and score before mortality.

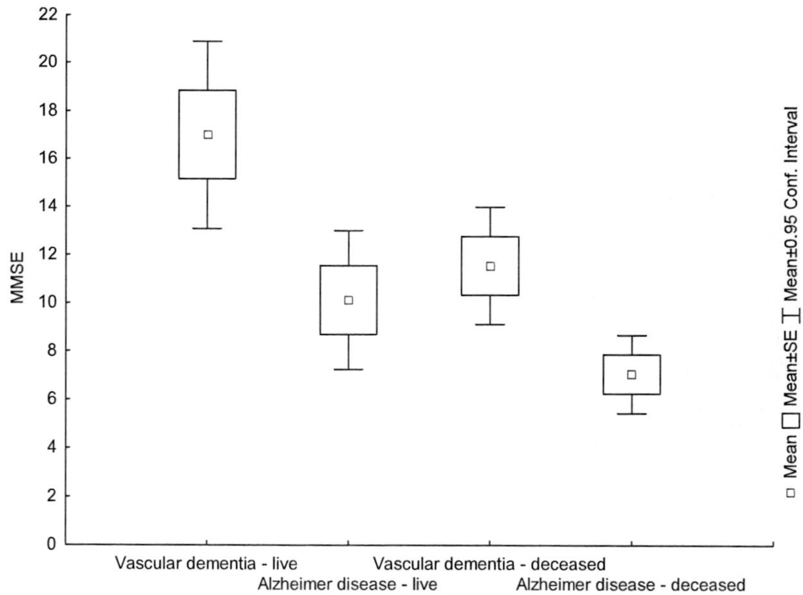

Figure 2. MMSE score within groups of patients defined by their diagnosis and mortality.

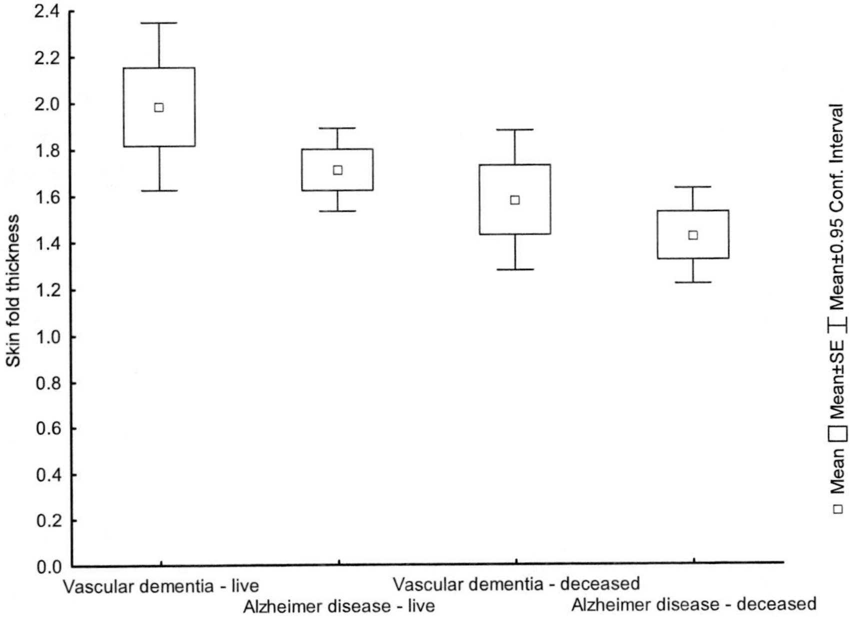

Figure 3. Skin fold thickness within groups of patients defined by their diagnosis and mortality.

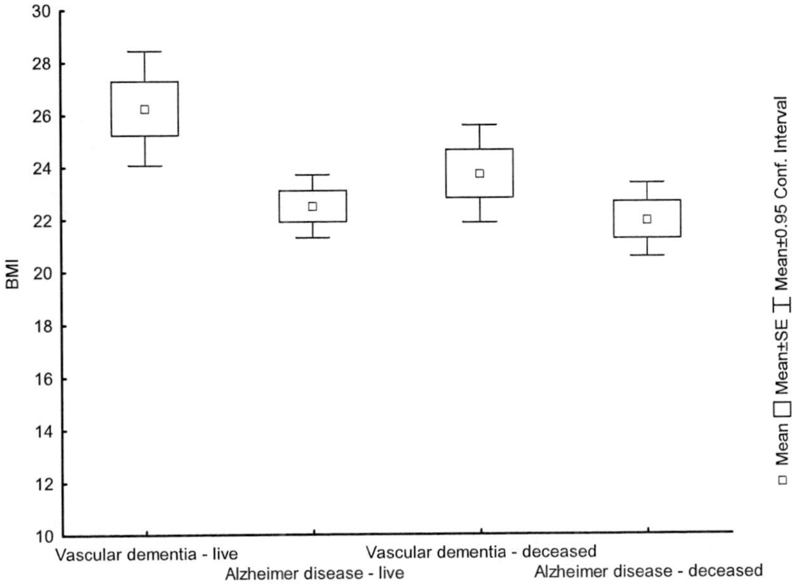

Figure 4. BMI within groups of patients defined by their diagnosis and mortality.

The energy intake correlated significantly with the values of the MMSE ($r=0.188$, $p<0.05$) as well as MNA ($r=0.256$, $p<0.05$), which suggests that the value of MNA can be a good indicator of voluntary food intake also in patients suffering from dementia. The correlation between MMSE and the food intake (energy) indicates that the food intake relates to the patients' mental state and the quality of life.

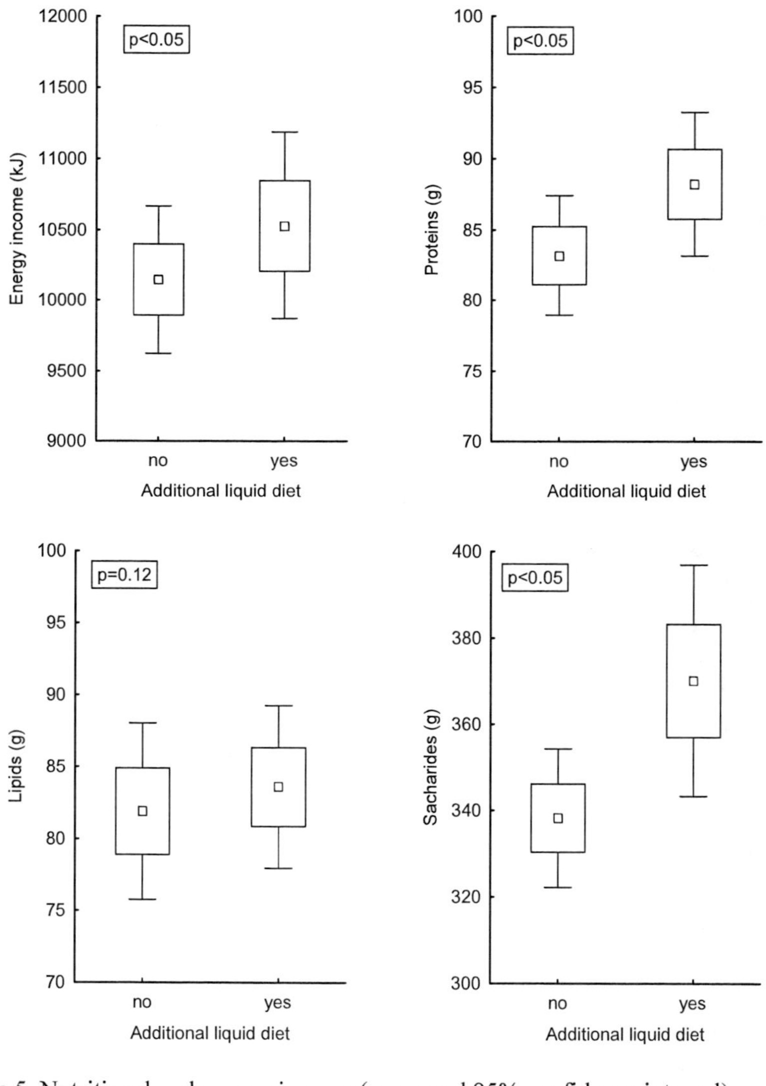

Figure 5. Nutritional and energy income (mean and 95% confidence interval) according to nutritional support.

Using retrospective time series analysis of the evaluated parameters categorized according to the patients' diagnosis and their potential mortality, a significant decrease in the MNA was discovered (Kruskall-Wallis ANOVA p=0.005) and MMSE (Kruskall-Wallis ANOVA p=0.004) were apparent in AD patients during the last three months of life. The same results were also obtained for the skin fold thickness.

Concerning the food components, the intake of proteins and carbohydrates was significantly higher in AD patients than in VD patients. No differences were found in the consumption of lipids.

Influence of Nutritional Support

The patients with AD who received a supplementary liquid diet had a constantly higher energy as well as protein intake. This is apparent from the analysis of the total nutrition intake. In spite of a slight decrease in the voluntary food intake in the supplemented group it can be concluded that nutritional supplements given to AD patients in the form of liquid diet led to a real increase in food intake (figure 5).

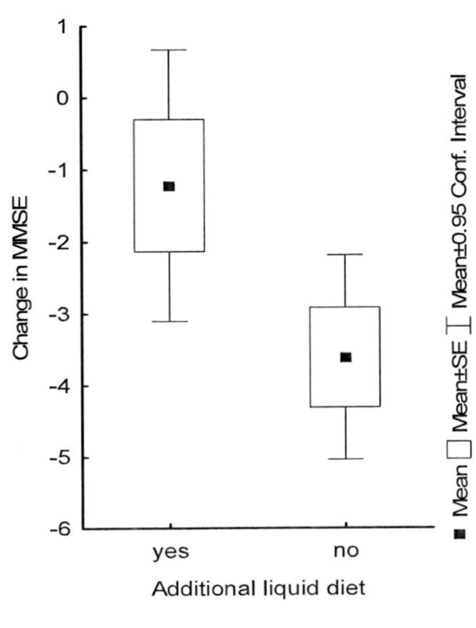

Figure 6. Change in MMSE parameter between first year (no sipping in this part of study) and the rest of study according to nutritional support of patients.

There was a decrease in the MMSE values in the group of AD patients without nutritional support within the study period. Nutritional support given in the form of food supplements averted this decrease. The difference was statistically significant (Kruskal Wallis ANOVA, p=0.024, figure 6).

However, no significant difference was found between the patients with and without nutritional support as far as survival analysis is concerned (Figure 7). We can thus conclude whereas survival is not influenced, the quality of life was significantly improved.

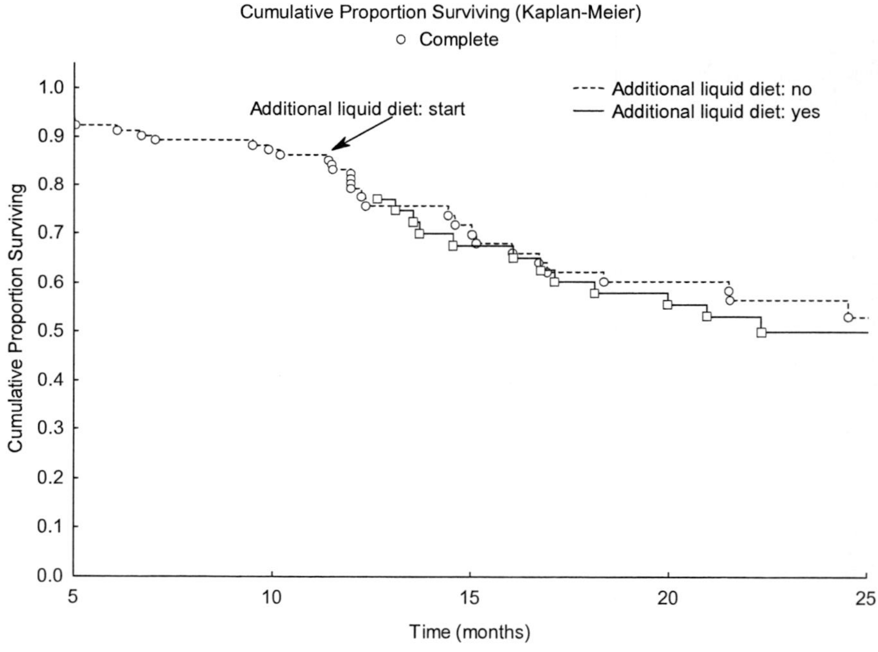

Figure 7. Comparison of survival of patients with Alzheimer disease and with and without nutritional support.

Discussion

To our knowledge, the relationship between the mental state, the state of nutrition and nutritional support in monitored long–term in individuals with AD, has not yet been described.

The relation between malnutrition and the risk of death in patients with AD has been described in a study that monitored 666 patients with AD in a time span of 6 years [5]. Each negative change in the phase of the AD was connected to a decrease in body weight (of about 1 kg). This finding supports the present finding that a decrease in body weight is linked to the progress of the disease. If a decrease in weight greater than 5% occurred within a year, it signified a great probability of death. On the other hand, an increase in weight lowered the risk of mortality [4]. Previous studies have dealt mainly with spontaneous food intake and their results tend to be controversial.

Although the relationship between the AD and the patients' weight loss has already been known for a long time, the aetiology of this relation is unknown [14, 15].

The lower food intake may play an important role in the body weight loss in AD patients. This can be related to the decline in cognitive function, the decrease of motivation, appetite and subsequent low food intake. The correlation between the reduction of the temporal cortex thickness and the changes in the limbic system, which determine appetite and food intake motivation, as well as the correlation of the medium temporal lobus (MTC) with BMI [10].support this view. Each negative change in the course of AD was correlated to a decrease in body weight (by about 1 kg), thereby implying to the connection between the decrease in body weight with the progress of AD [4].

A decline in physical exercise and muscle atrophy can also play a role in the body weight loss in AD patients. Reduction of physical activity, however, can occur as a common feature in both AD and VD patients and it therefore does not explain the aetiology of malnutrition in AD patients. Moreover AD patients are frequently physically active. We did not observe a lower energy intake in the AD patients than in the vascular dementia patients during our long-term study. In spite of this finding the nutrition status (expressed as BMI and other nutritional indicators) was lower in AD patients than in the patients with VD. It seems therefore that the gradual and progressive weight loss and development of malnutrition in AD is neither directly connected to the decrease of energy intake, nor to the decrease of physical activity [16].

The development of malnutrition in AD was obvious, in spite of the energy intake having been comparable to the energy intake of the patients with vascular dementia. An increase of energy expenditure or a change of the metabolic activity with an acceleration of catabolism may play a role in this progressive loss of weight. Some authors have reported a higher energy expenditure in AD patients and also showed that energy intake necessary for the maintenance of their body weight in a time span of 10 weeks was higher in these subjects (1626 vs. 1341 kcal, $p < 0.011$) [17] ;

similar results were obtained also by other authors [18,19]. On the other hand, others did not observe similar increase of energy expenditure in patients with Alzheimer's disease, in spite of more rapid loss of body weight than in the control subjects [20]. A correlation was also found between the amount of muscle mass and the energy intake as well as energy expenditure in AD patients. [21]

The development of malnutrition can also be connected to changes in the tissue metabolism, state similar to tumour cachexia, and possibly also to the metabolism of some vitamins [22, 23, 24, 25]. According to our results nutrition support not only improves nutrient intake but also slows down the progress of dementia and probably improve the quality of life of AD patients. This was confirmed by our findings in which we observed a slowing down of the deterioration of mental functions in those patients who received nutritional support. It is evident from our clinical experience that the energy need of AD patients may require 50-80 kcal/kg and day, to avoid a loss of body weight in some patients. [26]

An unfavourable state of some MNA and MMSE components was found in our study in patients with AD in spite of their lower age and their lower death rate than in the case of VD patients. Furthermore, when including the time aspect of the monitoring of the patients in the analysis, we found a significant decline of some MNA and MMSE components in the group of patients with AD, and without nutritional support, and also in the group of deceased AD patients.

Those AD patients disease who died in the course of our study showed a significant decline in their MNA and MMSE results during the last three months of their lives. This decline was not found in any other group of patients. Although the stated parameters are not direct indicators of malnutrition (as opposed to BMI [10] or the skin fold thickness), they are significantly linked to the food intake. The nutritional support of the Alzheimer's disease patients carried out in our study by liquid supplements was associated with an improved mental state as expressed using MMSE. This nutritional support can have a positive influence on the mental state of the patients with Alzheimer's disease and can slow down the progress of this disease. Although the survival of patients was not influenced by administered dose of additional liquid diet in this study, from our clinical experience on another patients with high dose of liquid diet it seems that also lifespan can be influenced; nevertheless these results are not statistically significant.

Acknowledgments

This study was supported by the Grant of the Ministry of Health of the Czech Republic XD/7964-3. The Czech Government had no role in the design of the study; the data collection, analyses or interpretation; or in the decision to publish the manuscript.

The work should be attributed to the Department of Psychiatry, Faculty of Medicine, Masaryk University, Brno, Czech Republic.

References

[1] Maurer K, Volk S, Gerbaldo H. Auguste D and Alzheimer's disease. *The Lancet* 1997; 349: 1546-1549.

[2] European commission. Alzheimer disease and other dementias *http://ec.europa.eu/health/ph_information/dissemination/diseases/alzheimer_en.htm 2005.*

[3] Finley B. Nutritional needs of the person with Alzheimer's disease: practical approaches to quality care. *J Am Diet Assoc* 1997; 97: S177-80.

[4] White H, Pieper C, Schmader K. The association of weight change in Alzheimer's disease with severity of disease and mortality: a longitudinal analysis. *J Am Geriatr Soc* 1998; 46: 1223-7.

[5] White H, Pieper C, Schmader K. The association of weight change in Alzheimer's disease with severity of disease and mortality: a longitudinal analysis. *J Am Geriatr Soc,* 1998;46:1223-7

[6] ICD-10 The ICD-10 Classification of mental and behavioural disorder. *Diagnostic criteria for research.* Work Health Organization Geneva, 1993, 248 p.

[7] Molsa PK, Paljarvi L, Rinne JO, Rinne UK, Sako E. Validity of clinical diagnosis in dementia: a prospective clinicopathological study. *J Neurol Neurosurg Psychiatry* 1985; 48: 1085-90.

[8] Cockrell JR, Folstein MF. Mini Mental State Examination (MMSE). *Psychopharmacology* 1988; 24: 689-692.

[9] Sunderland T, Hill JL, Mellow AM, Lawlor BA, Gundersheimer J, Newhouse PA, Grafman JH. Clock drawing in Alzheimer's disease: A novel measure of dementia severity. *Journal of the American Geriatrics Society* 1989; 37: 725-729.

[10] Galanos AN, Piper CF, Cornoni-Huntley JC, et al. Nutrition and function. Is there a relationship between body mass index and the functional capabilities of community-dwelling elderly? *J Am Geriatr Soc* 1994; 42: 368-73.

[11] McGee M, Jensen GL. Mini Nutritional Assessment (MNA): Research and Practice in the Elderly. *Nestle Nutrition Workshop Series Clinical & Performance Programme, vol 1*, edited by Hellas B, Garvey PJ, Guigoz Y 1999, S Karger AG, Basel, Switzerland. pp 195. Nutricom Software, Version 2.1, copyright (c) 2001 Nutricom

[12] StatSoft Inc. STATISTICA (data analysis software system), version 7. *www.statsoft.com* 2004.

[13] Wolf-Klein GP, Silverstone FA. Weight loss in Alzheimer's disease: an international review of the literature. *Int Psychogeriatr* 1994; 6: 135-42.

[14] Du W, DiLuca C, Growdon JH. Weight loss in Alzheimer's disease. *J Geriatr Psychiatry Neurol* 1993; 6: 34-8.

[15] Guyonnet S, Nourhashemi F, Ousset PJ, de Glisezinski I, Riviere D, Albarede JL. Vellas B Alzheimer's disease and nutrition. *Rev Neurol* (Paris) 1999; 155: 343-9.

[16] Wolf-Klein GP, Silverstone FA, Lansey SC, Tesi D, Ciampaglia C, O'Donnell M, Galkowski J, Jaeger A, Wallenstein S, Leleiko NS. Energy requirements in Alzheimer's disease patients. *Nutrition* 1995; 11: 264-8.

[17] Wolf-Klein GP, Silverstone FA, Levy AP. Nutritional patterns and weight change in Alzheimer patients. *Int Psychogeriatr* 1992; 4: 103-18.

[18] Spindler AA, Renvall MJ, Nichols JF, Ramsdell JW. Nutritional status of patients with Alzheimer's disease: a 1-year study. *J Am Diet Assoc* 1996; 96: 1013-8.

[19] Niskanen L, Piirainen M, Koljonen M, Uusitupa M. Resting energy expenditure in relation to energy intake in patients with Alzheimer's disease, multi-infarct dementia and in control women. *Age Ageing* 1993; 22: 132-7.

[20] Dvorak RV, Poehlman ET. Appendicular skeletal muscle mass, physical activity, and cognitive status in patients with Alzheimer's disease. *Neurology* 1998; 51: 1386-90.

[21] Riviere S, Birlouez-Aragon I, Nourhashemi F, Vellas B. Low plasma vitamin C in Alzheimer patients despite an adequate diet. *Int J Geriatr Psychiatry*, 1998;13:749-54

[22] Peskind ER. Pharmacologic approaches to cognitive deficits in Alzheimer's disease. *J Clin Psychiatry*, 1998;59 (Suppl.9):22-7.

[23] Pitchumoni SS, Doraiswamy PM. Current status of antioxidant therapy for Alzheimer's Disease. *J Am Geriatr Soc*, 1998;46:1566-72.

[24] Renvall MJ, Spindler AA, Ramsdell JW, Paskvan M. Nutritional status of free-living Alzheimer's patients. *Am J Med Sci*, 1989;298:20-7.

[25] Navrátilová M, Sobotka L, Hamrová E, Feketová J, Češková E. Etiologie malnutrice u pacientů s demencí - srovnání pacientů s Alzheimerovou chorobou a vaskulární demencí v multicentrické studii. *Psychiatrie*, Praha: Tigis; 7: 34-34. ISSN 122-7579. 2003 (In Czech).

In: Malnutrition: Risk Factors … ISBN: 978-1-62100-351-9
Editor: J.B. Knudsen

Chapter 7

RELATIONSHIP OF THE BLOOD PRESSURE AND NUTRITIONAL STATE OF THE PATIENTS WITH ANOREXIA NERVOSA AND BULIMIA NERVOSA: THE STUDY OF 117 PATIENTS IN THE 5 YEARS STUDY

Miroslava Navrátilová[1], Jiří Jarkovský[2], Jana Tůmová[3], Michaela Hamrová[4], Lubos Sobotka[5] and Brian Leonard[6]

[1] Department of Psychiatry, Medical Faculty Masaryk University and Faculty Hospital, Brno
[2]Institute of Biostatistics and Analyses, Masaryk University Hospital, Brno
[3]Dpt.of Clinical Biochemistry, Masaryk University Hospital, Brno
[4]Dpt.of Clinical Nutrition, St.Anna Hospital, Brno
[5] Gerontometabolic Clinic, University Hospital Hradec Kralove, Charles University, Czech Republic ,
[6]Pharmacology Dpt., National University of Ireland, Galway, Ireland

RATIONALE

Anorexia nervosa and bulimia nervosa are primary psychiatric diseases, which can be characterized by food intake problems.

Recorded history of eating disorders extends into the distant past. Starvation, receiving a reduced amount of food or modified diet has been part of many religious ceremonies and rituals, acts of protest or response to poor living conditions. Already in the 2nd century, Galen described the first symptoms of anorexia nervosa. In 12th to 15th century women starved to silence their sinful body and claimed to be a saint. In the 16th century, however, these women were alleged to be possessed by the devil, and women were victimized by the church officials. The turning point occurred in connection with the fashion trend in 1908, when P. Poiret, the Parisian fashion designer, introduced the unprecedented trend of clothing - the female body was shone through the dress. Since that time began to grow a variety of low-fat and low-saccharine diets, leading to leaner body especially the female body. In 1967, the model Twiggy (41 kg / 170 cm) appeared on the cover of fashion magazine Vogue. In 1970 the Swedish psychiatrist S. Theander warns of ominous rise in eating disorders - about 70% of American families buy low-calorie food. And ever slimmer girls win title of Miss America. The first special facility for patients with eating disorders was established in 1979. In 1987 anorexia nervosa and bulimia nervosa were declared by the WHO as important issue for the world's population. Since 1990, preventive and supportive programs for eating disorders are announced and the public is dissatisfied with excessive idealisation of emaciation and drastic dietary measures. Primary psychiatric illness is finally understood as a disease with very serious physical consequences - the result is a physical adaptation to prolonged fasting of organism with all the consequences, including the significant reduction of hormonal and immune activity.

These are called "autocannibalism", when organism consumes its own tissues and organs to survive. Physical complications, mainly cardiovascular and pulmonary, including disease of parenchymatous organ, unfortunately, can be lethal in approx. 25-35 percent. The mean length of survival is 33 years in these patients.

These statistical data include all deaths of the patients with eating disorders including influence of drug abuse like psychotropic drugs, laxatives, diuretics, thyroid hormones and alcohol. The deaths are also caused by suicide which is more frequent in bulimia nervosa.

Lack of criticism and poor compliance to the treatment are characteristic features of these diseases. Anorexia nervosa and bulimia nervosa are complicated also by subsequent malnutrition, primary or secondary amenorrhea and serious hormonal and immune malfunction. BMI of these severely malnourish patients is 10 – 16 kg/ m^2.

ANOREXIA NERVOSA

Anorexia nervosa is a form of restrictive eating disorders and is characterized by reducing the weight, which is deliberately induced and maintained. It is expressed by the specific psychopathology - fear of fatness. Patients have compulsive and obsidian thoughts to reduce their body weight [Picture 1]. The disease is also accompanied by the potential abuse of these substances – i.e. laxatives, diuretics and other drugs such as thyroid hormones, emetics and others; alcohol abuse is also possible especially in bulimia nervosa patients. Furthermore, we see various forms of self-harm, which thus exacerbate somatic condition and complicate treatment. Even with very intelligent girls, often higher education students, as we discovered they may infect peripheral or central vein even their own applications, such as tea through the venous catheter, disconnection of infusion sets and handling. This can lead to sepsis, which was not possible to unambiguously identify agents and to determine the antibiotic treatment. Many times we were forced to suppress sepsis and administer a combination of two or more antibiotics for a long time and prolong the period of hospitalization. The patient was thus in a state of serious life-threat with significant ongoing protein catabolism.

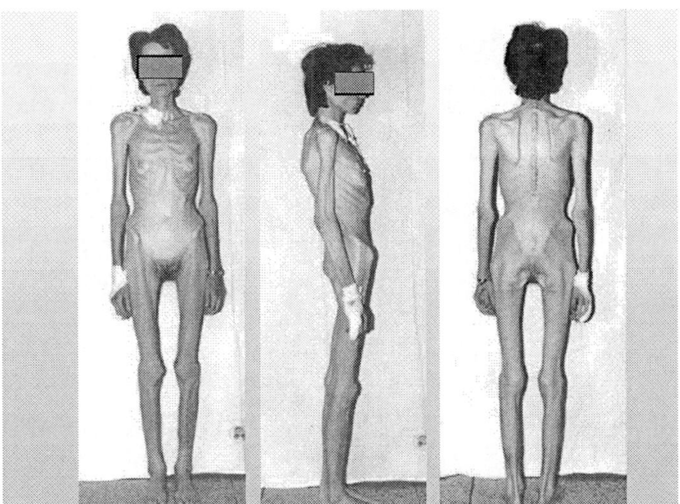

Picture 1. The patient with anorexia nervosa, hospitalized at the Intensive Care Unit Department of Psychiatry, Medical Faculty Masaryk University and Faculty Hospital Brno.

Bulimia Nervosa

Bulimia nervosa is the "ejection" form of eating disorders. According to statistics, this diagnosis is more common than the pure form of anorexia nervosa. According to our experience are both represented approximately equally in diagnosis and also very often both pathological entities - anorexia and bulimia are interconnected. The disease is characterized by repeated and uncontrollable seizures of large quantities of food intake, which is usually rich in calories. After a period of overeating the following occurs in patients: stomach fullness, bloating, pyros and other difficulties in gastrointestinal tract that are accompanied by feelings of depression and guilt. In a very short time period followed by compensational behavior when the patient tries to excessive amounts of ingested food to get rid of disability: they do so frequently by induced vomiting or use of laxatives. According to the information from our patients overeating is intentional, those sick already know in advance that the food they eat they soon regurgitate. They use a variety of practices, such as previous consumption of large quantities of grated carrots or other foods with a high content of residual substances. Repeated vomiting leads to electrolyte disturbances and other somatic complications. As mentioned in the introduction to this section , bulimia nervosa often occurs simultaneously with anorexia nervosa, or gradually develops for several months or years after its inception.

Comparison of anorexia nervosa and bulimia nervosa

	Anorexia nervosa	Bulimia nervosa
The incidence	1% (approximately 50% of women not dieting)	1-3%
Men Women	4% 96%	1% 99%
Frequent episodes of eating	rare	frequent
Vomiting	may be, sometimes frequent	regular
Use laxatives	frequent	frequent
Tendency to suicide	can occur	frequent
Body weight	regularly low	normal, reduced and increased
Abuse drugs	less frequent	frequent
Abuse alkohol	less frequent	frequent
Socio-economic layer	middle and upper	middle and higher
Cooperation	very little (so-called cooperation)	greater than MA
Mortality	resulting malnutrition	the result of electrolyte imbalance

Epidemiology

The disease is characteristic for developed countries. In third world countries is the death from the consequences of poverty and malnutrition or due to food shortage is typical, not due to anorexia nervosa or bulimia. For eating disorders malnutrition is the result of psychiatric illness. This is supported by the fact that we talk about the fact that approximately 50% of women in developed countries holds continuously or at short intervals in a diet.– The prevalence of anorexia nervosa in adolescents girls and young women is 1%, the disease occurs, according to our experience in the Center for Metabolism and nutrition disorders of the total number of patients at 96 per cent for women and four per cent for men. It affects mainly higher socio-economic layer, i.e. families with greater financial backing and a higher, mostly university graduates.– Bulimia nervosa occurs in about 1-3% of young women. For students of secondary schools and universities is the occurrence slightly higher. For men, the disease occurs in about ten times less frequently than in women. Although most patients have normal or reduced body weight, some patients may have a history and overweight.The data come from economically developed countries as in poor countries is not possible to unambiguously diagnose the disease (lack of food, the struggle for survival, famine)

Social Factors

Aspect currently means success and beauty. This proves the media presentation of "perfect" characters and actresses models etc. Subject to this pressure, are especially young girls, who at this time want to become a model, actress, mannequin or otherwise successful woman. This supports the fact that they often suffered from an eating disorder and even some celebrities such as singer Karen Carpenter, the actress Audrey Hepburn, it was that Princess Diana was diagnosed with bulimia nervosa. Another cause is the desire for conformity in partnership life arising from the notion that obesity, even supposed, can destroy relationship.

Psychological and Psychodynamic Factors

Interaction in families where there are anorexia nervosa, are often dysfunctional, psychoanalysts emphasize the avoidance of sexuality and the role played by the inability to break away from the mother. Between parents and daughter often even before the outbreak of the disease comes to the stormy confrontation and exchange of views, which in addition, to social influences - the pressure on young women to be thin. The typical syndrome is then referenced to immature personality structure. Internal problem often lies in the very process of adolescence, in adulthood and sexual maturity.

Eating disorders are often found in girls where their families are increasingly talking about eating the body shapes – figure. Initially well-intentioned efforts to reduce food intake by the patient can gradually leads up to the states of starvation with amenorrhea, and the girls at the time are often found even in pre-pubertal where sexual phase does not develop - or its development is braking. The patients particularly with anorexia nervosa have a fear of sexuality and returns to the infantile age with their thinking.

The personality features of the patients with bulimia nervosa often include impulsivity, anger, emotional lability, suicide attempts, alcohol abuse and petty theft (mostly food).

Diagnostic criteria for anorexia nervosa:

- Weight loss or weight gain of children lacking, leading to lower body weight by at least 15% compared to the normal or expected weight for age and height appropriate
- weight loss caused by avoiding foods, after which thickens
- perception of themselves as too fat with importunate fear of further weight gain
- Extensive endocrine disorder involving hypothalamic-pituitary-gonadal axis

Diagnostic criteria for bulimia nervosa:

- Repeated episodes of binge eating (at least twice a week for 3 months) during which they consumed in a short time, large amounts of food
- The constant preoccupation with food and strong urge to binge on food ingestion
- Patients attempting to face an eventual rise in body weight after eating a large amount of food some of the following manner:· provoked vomiting· provoked diarrhea· alternate periods of fasting· type anorectic medication, synthetic thyroid hormones or diuretics, if they occur in diabetic patients may try to omit insulin
- own feeling too thick with dogged by the fear of weight gain (usually resulting in underweight).

The common sign of the patiens with eating disorders is a certain degree of the serious malnutrition. The sense of our study was to find possible correlation between various degree of malnutrition and the value of the blood pressure and their clinical consequences in these patients.

The aims of our study were:

a) to describe the relation between the blood pressure and/or pulse and nutritional status in patients with anorexia nervosa and bulimia nervosa
b) to give a notice to the relation between blood pressure and s/u biochemical parameters, haematological parameters, anthropometric and dietetic parameters and hypothesis about the importance of blood pressure and pulse for identification of severe malnutrition.

METHODS

The dataset consist of 117 patients (39 bulimia nervosa, 55 anorexia nervosa, 22 mixed form), [Figure 1]. Most of the pacients were from 10 to 35 years old, [Figure 2]. Mean age of them is 25 years; women form 90.6% of the dataset, [Figure3].The patients are observed in long term study; the median of observations is 4, median follow up is 13.2 months, [Figure 4]

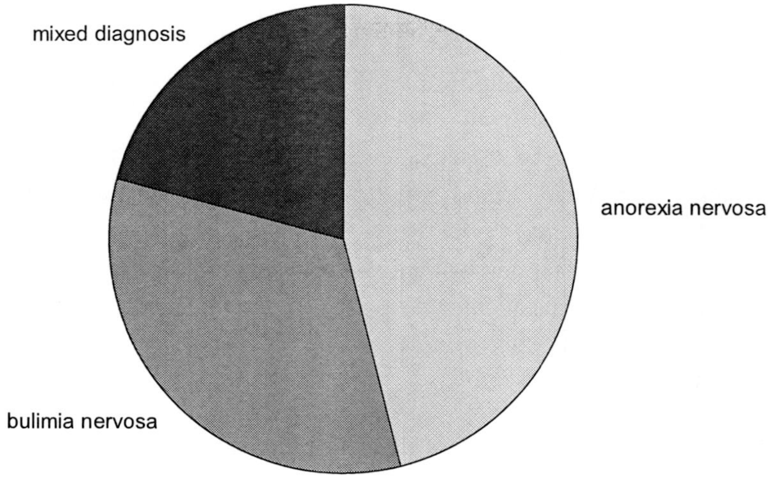

Figure 1. Diagnosis of the patients.

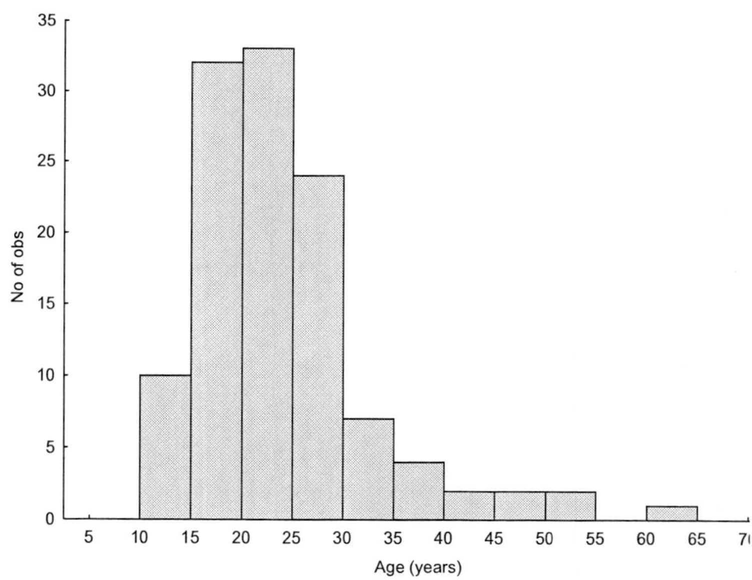

	Valid N	Mean	Median	Minimum	Maximum
Age (years)	117	24.6	23.0	11.0	61.0

Figure 2. Age structure of the patients.

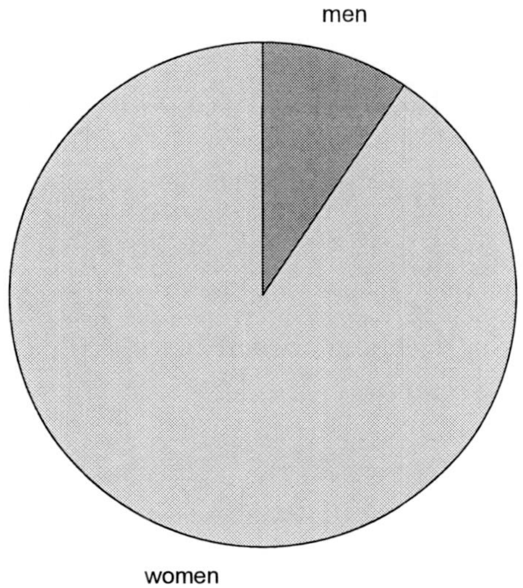

Figure 3. Sex structure of the patients.

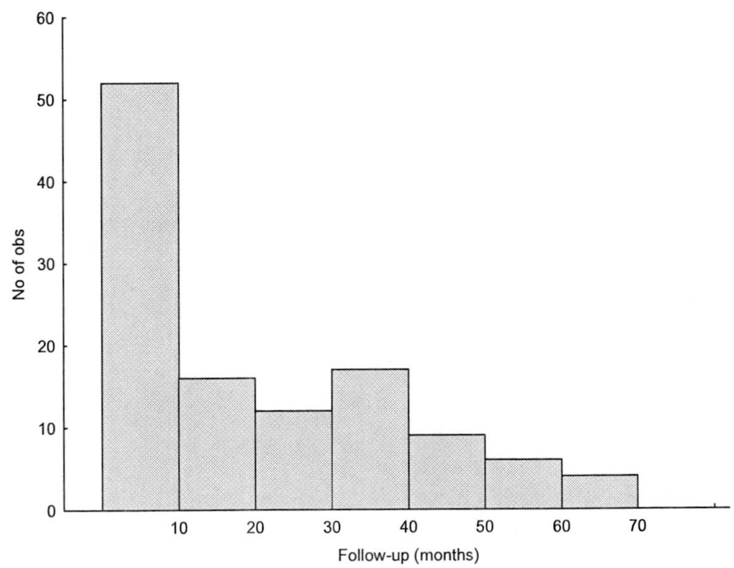

	Valid N	Mean	Median	Minimum	Maximum
Follow-up (months)	117	19.8	13.2	0.0	69.8

Figure 4. Follow up of the patients.

Input data: we did complex somatic and biochemical examination of each patient. Somatic state was examined at each control including ECG, blood pressure and heart rate, [Figure 9]. Contemporaneously with the values of blood pressure and pulse rate the following set of detailed parameters was observed during 3 working days and one whole weekend:

Anthropometric parameters

- Height, weight, BMI, arm circumference, calf circumference, total fat - BIA in %, kg [Figure 5]

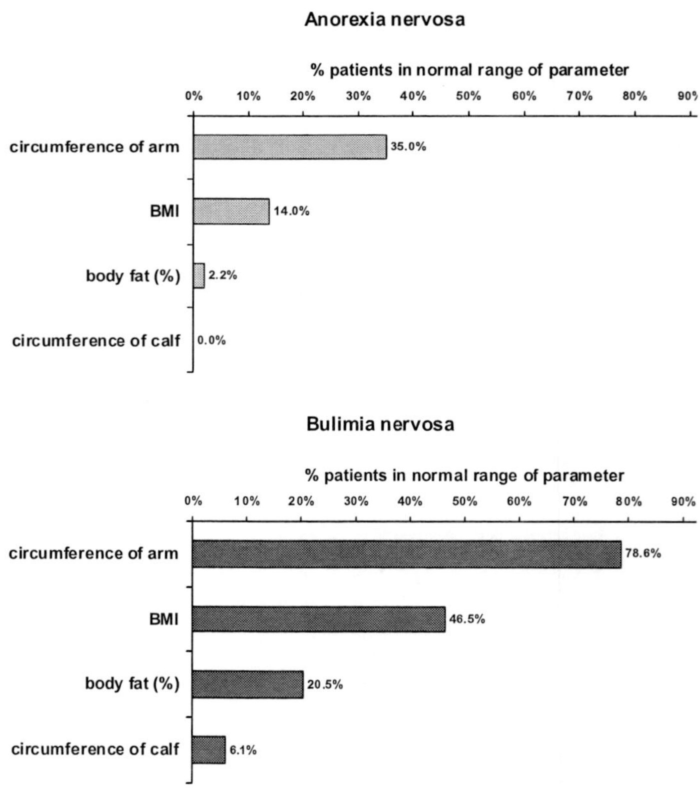

Muscle atrophy, reduction up to depletion of the fat tissue: no patient with anorexia nervosa had physiological circumference of calf during the study (in patients with bulimia nervosa it was only 6,1 percent)

Figure 5. Anthropometry parameters of patients in our study group.

Biochemical parameters

- Serum: glucose, urea, creatinine, uric acid, Na, K, Cl, Ca, Mg, P, Zn, Cu, Fe, Se, ALT, AST, GMT, LD, CK, amylase, lipase, cholesterol, HDL-cholesterol., LDL-cholesterol, triglycerides, transferin, albumin, prealbumin, total protein, thyroid hormones [Figure 6]
- Urinary output of – urea, creatinine , total nitrogen, Na, K, Cl, Mg, P, Zn, Cu, [Figure 7]

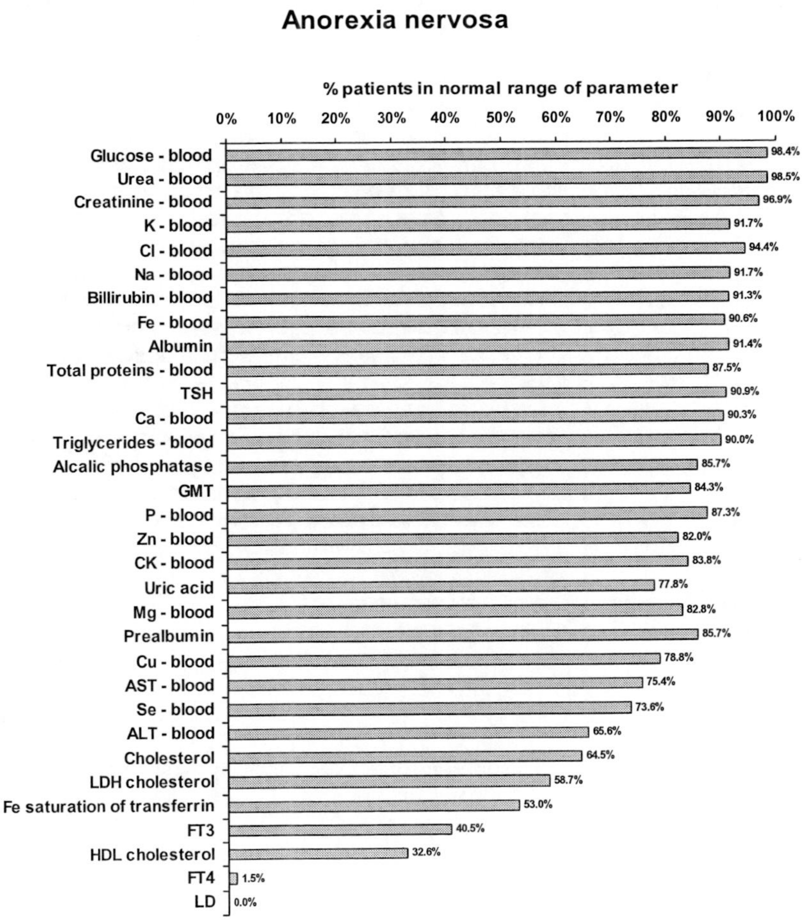

Figure 6. (continues).

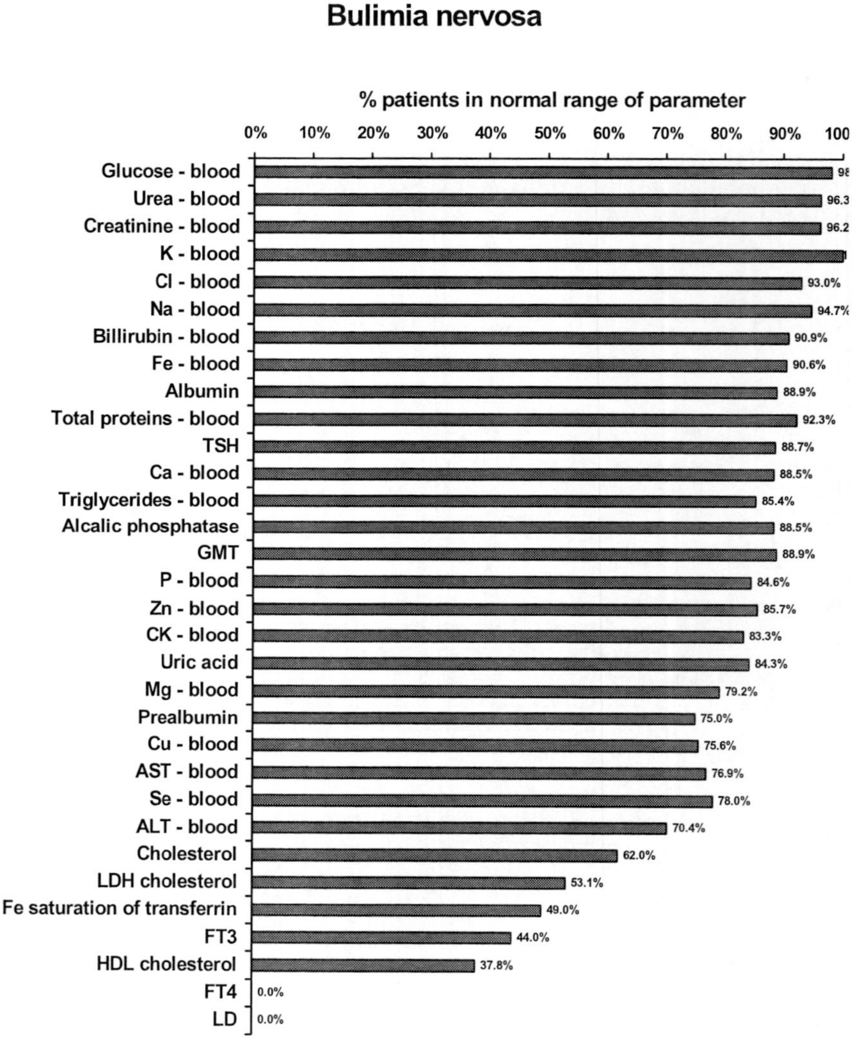

The rank of parameters according to % of patients in normal range of parameter is similar for anorexia and bulimia nervosa. The most disturbed parameters are FT4 and LD

Figure 6. Biochemical parameters of patients in our study group.

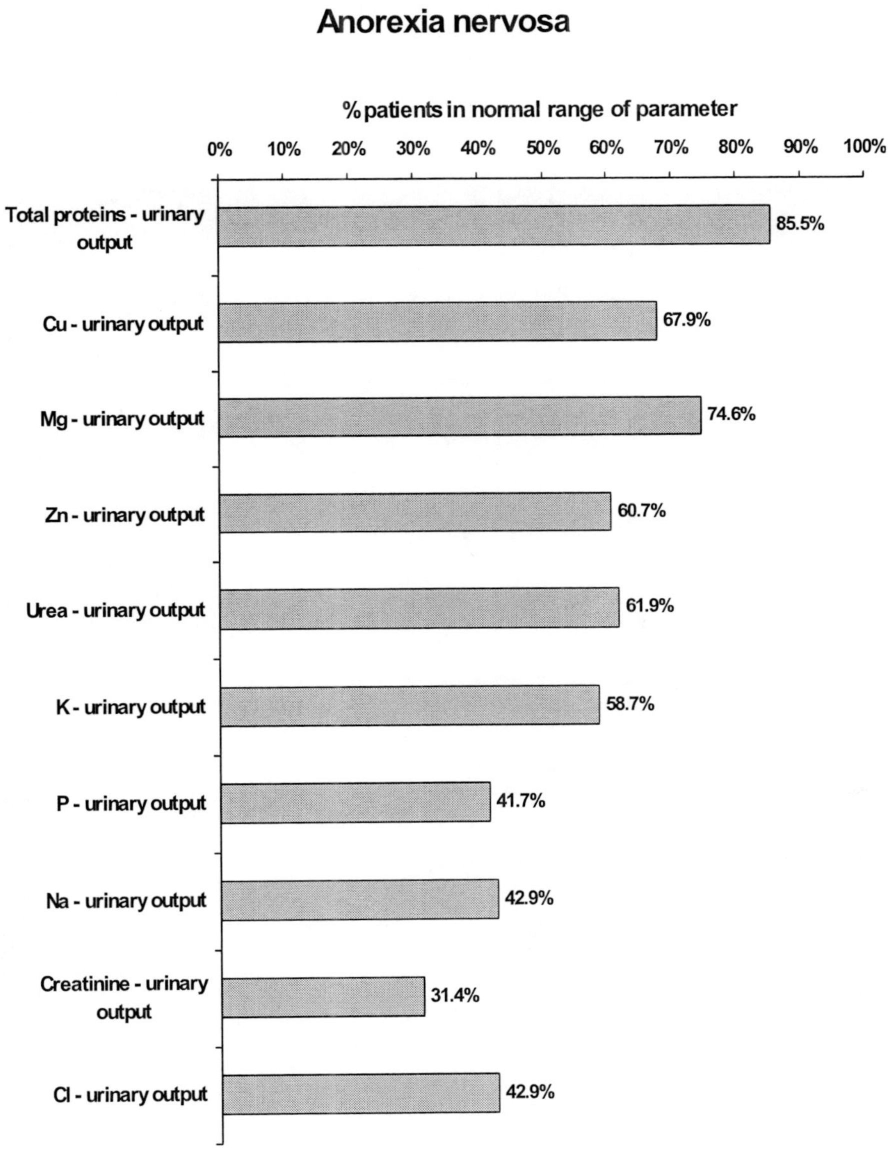

Figure 7. (continues).

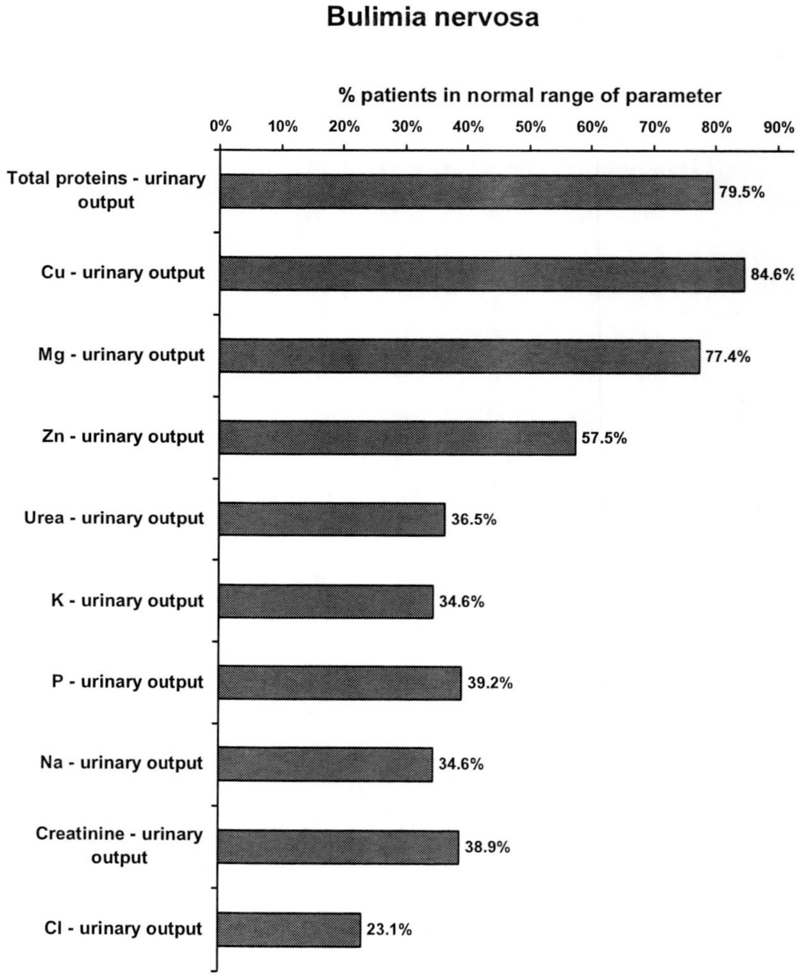

Some differences among patients with anorexia and bulimia nervosa can be found according to % of patients in normal range of parameter; namely for example urinary output of Cu, urea, K, Cl.

Figure 7. Urinary output of patients in our study group.

Hematological parameters

- Blood count + diff.

Dietetic parameters - food intake [Figure 8]

- The amount of macronutrients

- Intake of carbohydrate. fat, proteins during 3 working days and one weekend
- The amount of micronutrients
- Vitamins, electrolytes and trace elements

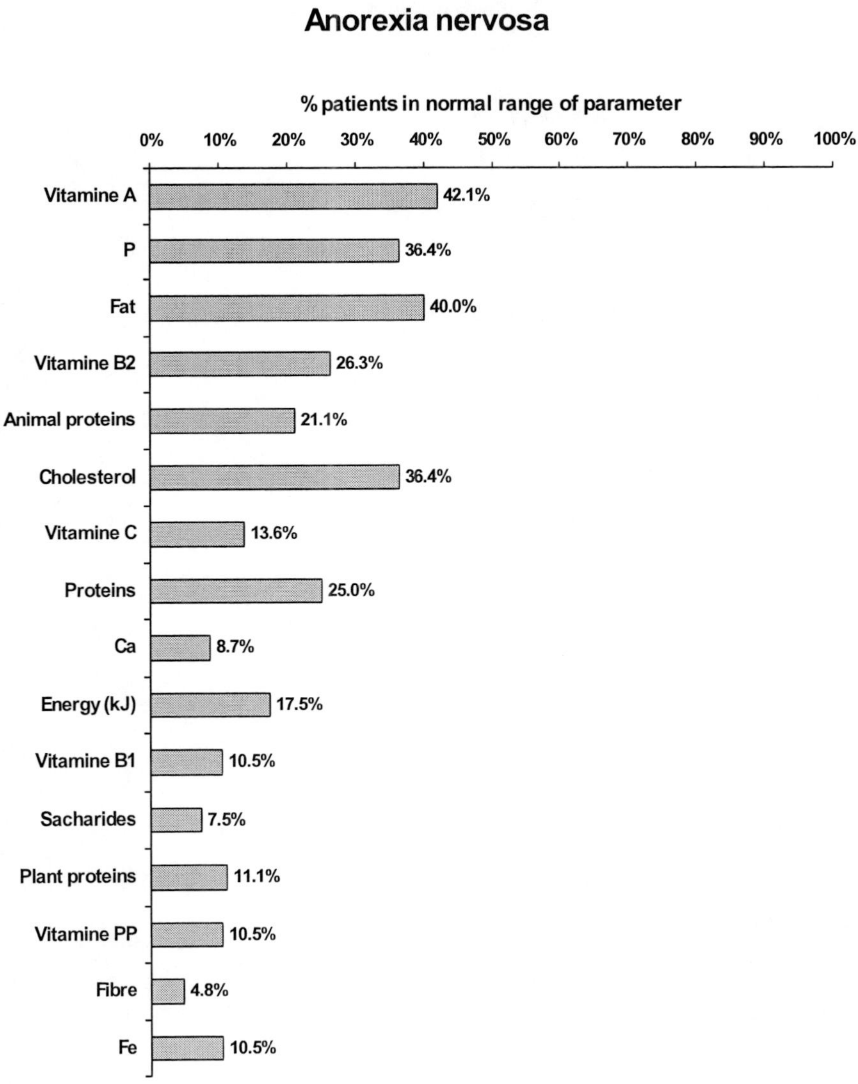

Figure 8. (continues).

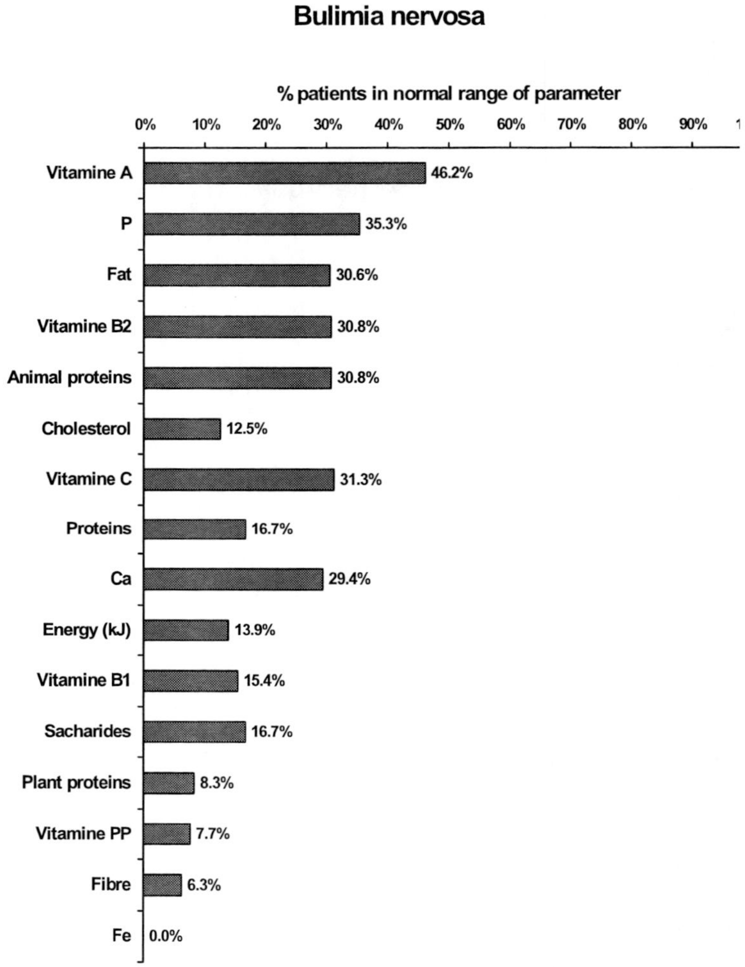

Some differences among patients with anorexia and bulimia nervosa can be found according to % of patients in normal range of parameter; namely for example cholesterol, vitamin C, proteins, Ca.

Figure 8. Food intake of patients in our study group.

To balance the different length of patients' observations, the analysis was computed on aggregated data; Spearman rank correlation coefficient was adopted for analysis of relationship between state of nutritional, biochemical, haematological, anthropometric and dietetic parameters and blood pressure and pulse. Principal component analysis was adopted for the visualization of the whole picture of parameters relationships.

RESULTS

The median value of diastolic and systolic blood pressure is 67 and 108 mm Hg respectively, these values should be considered as mark of abnormality of these parameters. The parameters of blood pressure and pulse are in statistically significant relationship to all parameters of patients' nutritional state (BMI, circumference of arm and calf, body fat etc.) and also to some biochemical parameters of their blood, [Table 1].

Table 1. Correlations between patients pulse, blood pressure and their nutritional and biochemical parameters (only parameters with significant correlation (in bold italic) with at least one of blood pressure or pulse parameters are shown)

	Systolic pressure	Diastolic pressure	Pulse
weight	***0.74***	***0.70***	***0.53***
BMI	***0.68***	***0.61***	***0.45***
circumference of arm	***0.61***	***0.48***	***0.38***
body fat (kg)	***0.48***	***0.40***	***0.27***
body fat (%)	***0.48***	***0.44***	***0.32***
detectable body fat	***0.43***	***0.39***	***0.32***
circumference of calf	***0.46***	***0.46***	***0.46***
S-Se	***-0.41***	***-0.36***	***-0.26***
S-GMT	***-0.28***	***-0.24***	***-0.34***
S-T3	***0.42***	***0.39***	***0.42***
S-CRP	***-0.31***	***-0.37***	-0.16
S-proteins	***0.24***	***0.29***	0.03
S-ALT	***-0.28***	***-0.25***	***-0.21***
sat.transf.(Fe)	***-0.28***	***-0.22***	-0.05
S-AST	***-0.26***	***-0.24***	***-0.27***
S-Cu	0.10	0.13	***0.28***
dU-Cl	***-0.24***	***-0.24***	-0.15
S-Mg	-0.11	-0.12	***-0.23***
S-TSH	***-0.21***	-0.15	-0.16
S-ALP	-0.10	***-0.21***	-0.12
S-urea	-0.13	***-0.21***	-0.07
S-prealbumin	0.20	0.25	***0.34***
dU-urea	-0.19	***-0.20***	-0.07

The parameters of blood pressure and pulse are in statistically significant relationship to all parameters of patients' nutritional state (BMI, circumference of arm and calf, body fat etc.) and also to some biochemical parameters of their blood.

Biochemical Parameters

We have found in our study group decrease of S-level of total protein, S-Cu and S-T3 with subsequent increase TSH (contribution of adaptation hormonal reduction within the secondary hypothyreosis) with statistically significant positive correlation of the value of the blood pressure and pulse rate (S-Cu). Moreover, decrease of the S-urea, S-urin acid, cholesterol, LDL-cholesterol level, S-Fe, sat.transf.(Fe) and decrease of transaminasis, which in the negative relationships with the blood pressure, esp. S-GMT, S-ALT, S-AST in the patients in the fore phase of realimentation. Surprisingly, by contrast the level of prealbumin and albumin did not have significant differences from physiological values, esp. in the patients with bulimia nervosa. However, each decrease of the level of S-prealbumin was connected with decrease of the blood pressure and of the pulse rate, which was in the correlation with a clinical state of the patients. The level of S-CRP did not differ significantly from physiological values in the both groups of patients; it was in clinical correlation with negative relationship which we have found between blood pressure and S-CRP. The plasma level of the trace elements surprisingly did not differ from physiological values, which is also in clinical correlation with negative relationship between blood pressure and S-Se.

Urinary outputs of electrolytes in 24hours were in both diagnoses significantly lowered in spite of the fact that S-levels did not differ significant from physiological values correlation with negative relationship of the blood pressure and S-Mg.

The level of electrolytes in urine correlated with the degree of metabolic consequences. Between the blood pressure and the level of dU-urea and dU-Cl was not the statistically significant positive correlation, we have found negative relationships, which could be connected with our clinical experience in patients with bulimia nervosa where we observe marked retention of dU-Cl in terms of bulimia episodes with almost physiological values of the blood pressure contrary with the patients with anorexia mentalis.

On the basis of these results it was possible to establish further treatment in correction of mineral and trace elements, including selection of parenteral or enteral substitution.

Diastolic blood pressure correlated significantly with BMI, Diastolic blood pressure correlated significantly with body fat, Diastolic blood pressure correlated significantly with arm circumference, Diastolic blood pressure correlated significantly with plasma Cu level. Diastolic blood pressure correlated significantly with plasma total protein and with level of plasma pre-albumin [Figure 11].

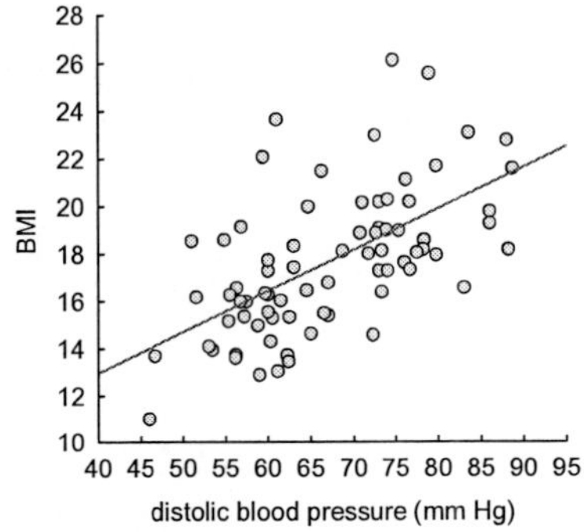

Diastolic blood pressure correlated significantly with BMI

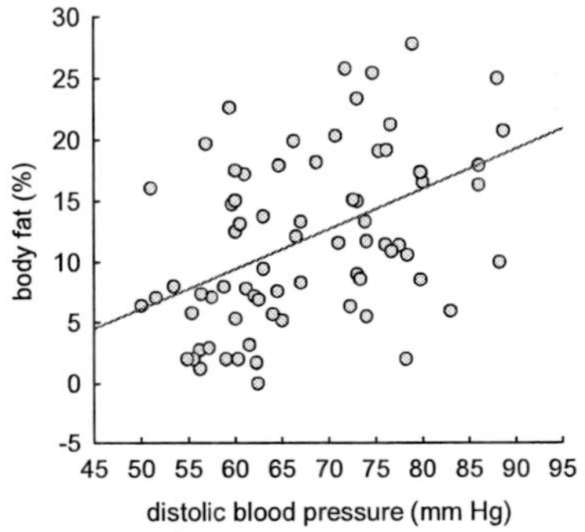

Diastolic blood pressure correlated significantly with body fat

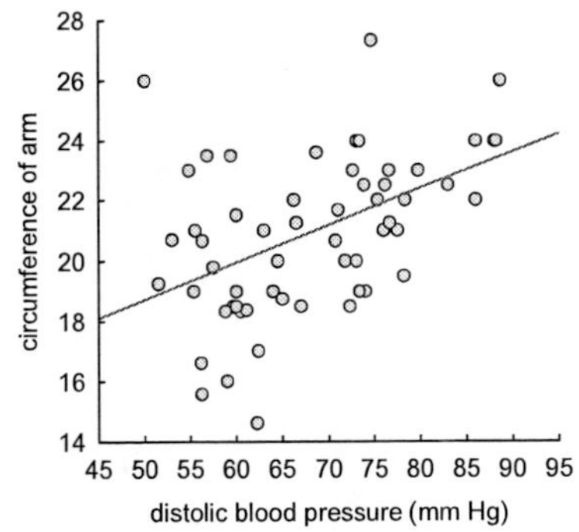

Diastolic blood pressure correlated significantly with plasma Cu level

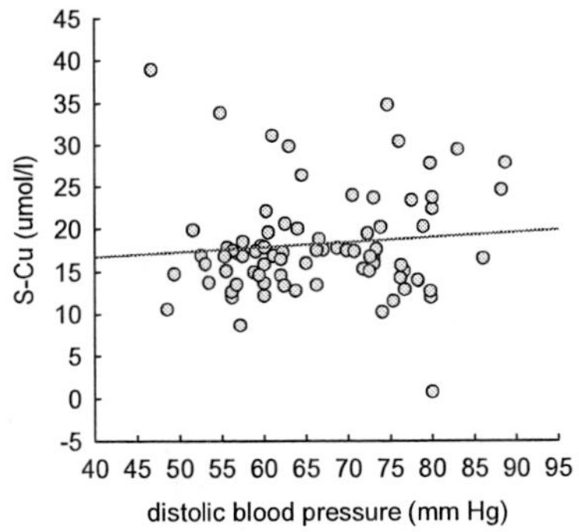

Diastolic blood pressure correlated significantly with arm circumference

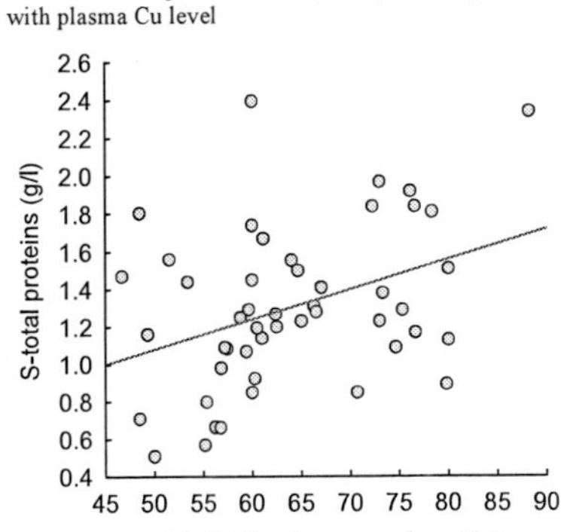

Diastolic blood pressure correlated significantly with plasma total protein

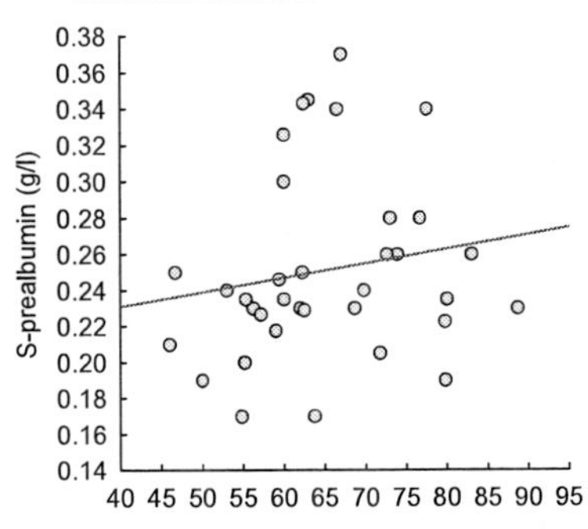

Diastolic blood pressure correlated significantly with level of plasma pre-albumin

Figure 11. Relationship of diastolic blood pressure and selected parameters of patients.

Statistically significant positive correlation between blood pressure and/or pulse and weight, BMI, circumference of arm, body fat (kg), body fat (%), detectable body fat, circumference of calf, S-T3, S-proteins, S-Cu and S-prealbumin were found. Negative relationships were found between blood pressure and/or pulse and S-Se, S-GMT, S-CRP, S-ALT, sat.transf.(Fe), S-AST, dU-Cl, S-Mg, S-TSH, S-ALP, S-urea and dU-urea, [Figure 10].

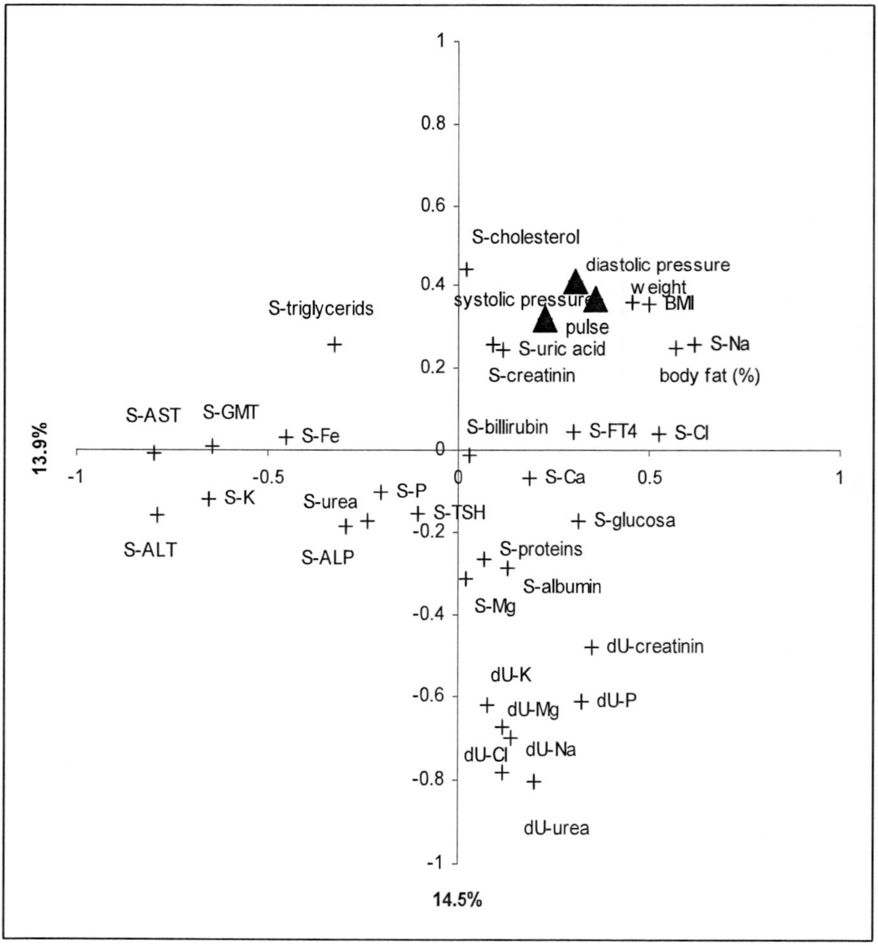

Figure 10. The figure shows position of blood pressure and pulse in factorial space of patients nutritional and biochemical parameters. Note the similar position of these parameters and parameters of nutritional state.

Diet

The analysis of the intake of food was in the correlation with a degree of malnutrition and it holds for both macro and micronutrients. Surprisingly we have found the marked reduction of protein and fibre intake in this type of patients, which in combination with protein catabolism deepened the protein malnutrition. It was in cross-correlation with anthropometric parameters and with the values of the blood pressure.

Anthropometry

Anthropometric parameters showed significant correlation with the values of blood pressure and pulse rate. The lower weight of the patients, esp. in the group with anorexia nervosa, correlated with the low values of the blood pressure. We have found muscle atrophy, reduction up to depletion of the fat tissue with statistically significant decrease of the values of the blood pressure and pulse rate, esp. in the patients with anorexia nervosa, whereas the body fat in physiological interval was only in 2.2 percent of the patients with anorexia nervosa. No patients with anorexia nervosa reached during five-year observation physiological circumference of calf (in patients with bulimia nervosa it was only 6.1 percent), whereas circumferences of arm and of the calf correlated with the decrease of the values of the blood pressure and pulse rate and these correlations were statistically significant.

CONCLUSIONS

Anorexia nervosa and bulimia nervosa are psychiatric disease with very serious somatic consequences. The patients with anorexia nervosa and bulimia nervosa suffer from various degree of malnutrition.

The relationship between the blood pressure and set of biochemical and nutritional parameters of patients was found with generally abnormal values of blood pressure in patients with anorexia nervosa and bulimia nervosa.

We found statistical significant changes in blood pressure and pulse rate in these patients which correlated significantly with degree of malnutrition and inflammatory reaction.

We can conclude that increase of body weight through correct realimentation could normalize values of blood pressure and its clinical consequences.

Monitoring of the changes in the blood pressure and heart rate could be simple and useful parameter signalising severity of malnutrition in bulimia and anorexia nervosa patients.

Disclosure of Interest

I declare that I do not have any affiliation with or financial interest in a commercial organisation that poses a conflict of interest

INDEX

D

E

F

G

H

I

J

K

L

M

N

O

P

Q

R

S

T

U

V

W

X

Y

Z